# Tone and Speech Eurythmy

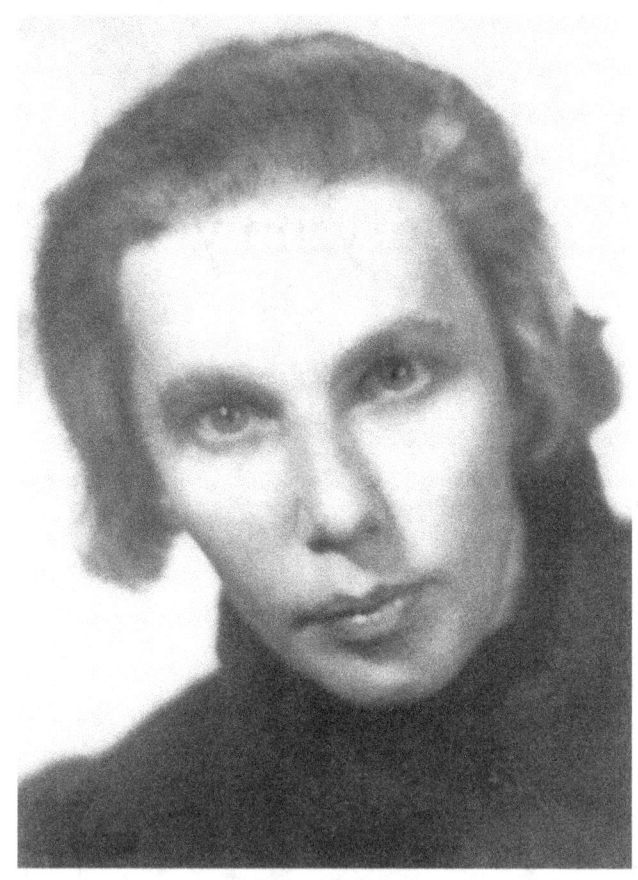

*Elena Zuccoli (1901–96)*
*by permission of Ingrid Braunschmidt*

# Tone and Speech Eurythmy

Elena Zuccoli

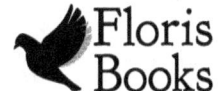

Translated by Dorothea Mier and Clifford Venho
Line drawing by Rosemarie Matthées (based on sketches by Elena Zuccoli)

First published in German as *Ton- und Lauteurythmie*
by Verlag Walter Keller, Dornach in 1997
First published in English by Floris Books, Edinburgh in 2023

© 1997 Estate of Elena Zuccoli
English translation © 2023 Floris Books

All rights reserved. No part of this book may be
reproduced in any form without written permission of
Floris Books, Edinburgh
www.florisbooks.co.uk

 Also available as an eBook

British Library CIP Data available
ISBN 978-178250-867-0

# Contents

| | |
|---|---|
| Foreword | 9 |
| 1. The First Impulse in 1915 | 13 |
| 2. Reawakened Interest in Tone Eurythmy | 27 |
| 3. The Birth of the First Eurythmy School | 31 |
| 4. The Christmas Conference 1923/24 | 43 |
| 5. New Foundations of Tone Eurythmy | 45 |
| 6. Tone Colours | 75 |
| 7. The Eurythmy Figures | 81 |
| 8. Speech Eurythmy | 91 |
| 9. Costumes | 107 |
| 10. Eurythmy Work with Marie Steiner | 113 |
| Notes | 119 |
| Bibliography | 123 |
| Index | 125 |

Beauty is not the divine in a sensory-real garment; no, it is the sensory-real in a divine garment. The artist does not bring the divine to earth by letting it flow into the world but by raising the world up to the sphere of the divine.
*Rudolf Steiner, 'Goethe as Father of a new Aesthetics' in* Art and Theory of Art, *p. 20.*

# Foreword

I first experienced Elena Zuccoli in 1970 when she was giving a course on Rudolf Steiner's indications for tone eurythmy. I was thrilled – it made so much sense and supported so much of what came later. She spoke out of her own experiences and was able to convey the mood of that time, making it so immediate. She had a very dynamic personality. Her eurythmy was very dramatic, and she was an inspiring teacher. She had flashing eyes, a lovely warm smile, and a deep chuckle.

Elena Zuccoli was born on November 14, 1901, in Milan, Italy. Her father was an Italian engineer, her mother a violinist from Finland. Both were anthroposophists. Her childhood was spent in both countries, and she later studied painting in Finland and music in Italy. In 1922 she joined the Eurythmy School in Stuttgart and participated in the Christmas Foundation meeting in 1923/24 where she gave a first solo performance.

She was asked by Marie Steiner to join the stage work at the Goetheanum, and so remained in Dornach after the Christmas Conference. She took part in the Speech Eurythmy Course in 1924 and taught tone eurythmy for about ten years at the Eurythmy School in Dornach under Isabelle de Jaager's direction.

From 1939 for about ten years she taught eurythmy and anthroposophy in Rome with Annie Heuser. She then took on the leadership of a newly created second stage group at the Goetheanum and founded her own Eurythmy School in Dornach.

At the age of seventy she stopped performing and my impression was that, through this, she became much freer. She stood very upright and was still teaching large courses into her nineties. She died in Arlesheim, Switzerland, on August 26, 1996.

This book, written at the end of her life, contains one gem after another. It is wonderful to have so many indications and to be able to refer back to them, refreshing my memory, but also for it to be available to those who did not have the chance to meet her. I am happy to finally make this available to the English-speaking world.

Dorothea Mier
September 2022

## *Acknowledgments*

We would like to thank the following organisations and people for their support: the Eurythmy Association of North America and the Melrose Pitman Fund for the North American work of the Performing Arts Section of the School of Spiritual Science for their generous grants that funded the translation and editing of this book; Floris Books for recognising the importance of this work and for making it available to all who seek it; and Melissa Lyons for her steadfast support and her generous contribution of time and effort to oversee the project.

Dorothea Mier and Clifford Venho

# 1

# The First Impulse in 1915

People have always asked how eurythmy began. This new art, encompassing the whole of the human being, has its origin in the spirit and was pre-ordained from the beginning of time in the plan of evolution.

Despite the endeavours of great artists such as Isadora Duncan, Mary Wigman, Alexander Sakharoff, and others, all that took place at the turn of the century to rejuvenate dance remained stuck in individual expressions of the soul. The efforts of the theosophist and dancer Rudolf Laban, who was the first to want to develop dance as a silent language, also did not bear fruit. They all felt the impulse of the time but remained fettered to the sensory element of nature. Their dance, like nature itself, carried death within it; that is, in the end, it led to mime-like movements, which should stand as a warning before us.

Rudolf Steiner raised dance to quite another level. He had the capacity to grasp the spiritual origins of the mobility of the human form (gestalt) and was able, through the *new* art of dance, to unite the physical body of the human being with the original forces out of which it was fashioned. Prior to this, dance arose out of old forces, but now something completely new could arise. The creative activity of the Logos could now reveal itself in the movements of the human being.

For some time, Rudolf Steiner had been looking for a suitable individual with whom he could explore the development of a new art of dance, a new art that would only find its fulfilment in the distant future.

Almost as in a fairy tale, a very young Lory Maier-Smits appeared in 1911. Who but she – with her endless devotion, persistence, strength, and love – could realise the birth of an art whose archetype is only to be found in the spirit? Eurythmy could not have had a more beautiful beginning.

Rudolf Steiner formed the lessons in such a way that he gave Lory Smits tasks and, only when necessary, indicated gestures himself. It was important to him that she learn to experience for herself and to grasp the gestures with feeling so that this new art would become completely her own.

For instance, she was to experience everything that happens when we walk, to experience with feeling all the variations of mood that can be expressed through walking. Furthermore, she was to acquaint herself with the laws of anatomy. She needed to sense with feeling how the sounds of speech can lead to different forms in space. This walking in space was accompanied by positions and movements of the arms. Gestures for the sounds of speech had not yet been given.

Why did Rudolf Steiner find it necessary for her to practice walking as well as feeling her way into space, without arm gestures, for almost a year? It becomes clear that through this kind of practising he wanted to awaken the experience of the fundamental forces that are necessary in order to practise the art of eurythmy.

There are two forces upon which eurythmy can build its foundation and take hold of the physical body in a meaningful way.

One force is the sense of balance in the human being, which allows us to differentiate between up and down in the broadest sense of the word. It has an expansive effect on the etheric, which allows us to integrate ourselves in space.[1]

The second force is quite different. It appears in early childhood, places us into the vertical and teaches us to walk. In every human being an unused, unconscious portion of this force of uprightness remains. This innocent, pure force, when it is later awakened, can become an organ that recognises the motif of our personal destiny. The force of uprightness is grasped in threefold walking through the sense of balance, which lives in the human being as the outcome of previous earthly lives:

> There is something that entails the exercise of a great many forces – the fact that human beings do not go about on all fours throughout life but at an early age acquire the faculty of *standing upright*. The forces enabling man to assume the vertical position are of such a nature that they inspire a quite special reverence in one who has penetrated into the spiritual world ...
> ... These forces that have been saved generally remain unheeded, but awareness of them can be promoted by practising a certain form of dance ... for a little less than a year now, certain groups of people among us have been working at Eurythmy, an art based on the principles of the movements of the etheric body.
> Eurythmy is nothing like ordinary gymnastics or dancing ... but the movements made are in complete accord with those of the etheric body. Through these free movements the human being will gradually discover and become aware of the forces that are still within him. Foundations are being created for the awakening of forces within the human being which will really enable him to see into the spiritual worlds stretching between his last death and his birth in the present life.[2]

To avoid any misunderstanding, it must be said that other forces activate the creation of the larynx, and that there is a third force that produces the capacity to think in the human being.

Eurythmy grew and developed during the time when the first Goetheanum was being built. On the stage of the carpentry shop in 1915, scenes from Goethe's *Faust* were performed in eurythmy: Easter Night, Ariel's scene, and Ascension. In the late summer of that same year, a second eurythmy course was given, despite the First World War. Prior to the course, many lectures had been given to the artists working on the Goetheanum, especially about music. Through these, Rudolf Steiner wanted to awaken an understanding for artistic creativity with newly emerging forms and colour, free of any naturalism.

After the Dionysian element in eurythmy had been developed in the previous years, the more cosmic side of the word was now dealt with. Thus, as a complement, the Apollonian element was added.

When we consider the sequence of themes in all of Rudolf Steiner's lectures, it is amazing how organically the one follows from the other, and we recognise the masterful grasp of spiritual economy in the way he artistically made a transition from one theme to the next. We can learn an endless amount from this.

It is striking how Rudolf Steiner prepares the new element of music (tone) eurythmy in 1915. In this course, he gave the Apollonian forms. The cosmic poem of his own creation entitled the *Twelve Moods,* as well as the *Dance of the Planets* and the satirical *Song of Initiation* were likewise practised and performed. The right inner mood thus arose in those present. This made it possible for him to introduce the new impulse of tone eurythmy. Both the Apollonian forms and the new poems bear the musical element – the Apollonian element in its inner logic and the *Twelve Moods* in its structure and in the new kind of speech that it created.

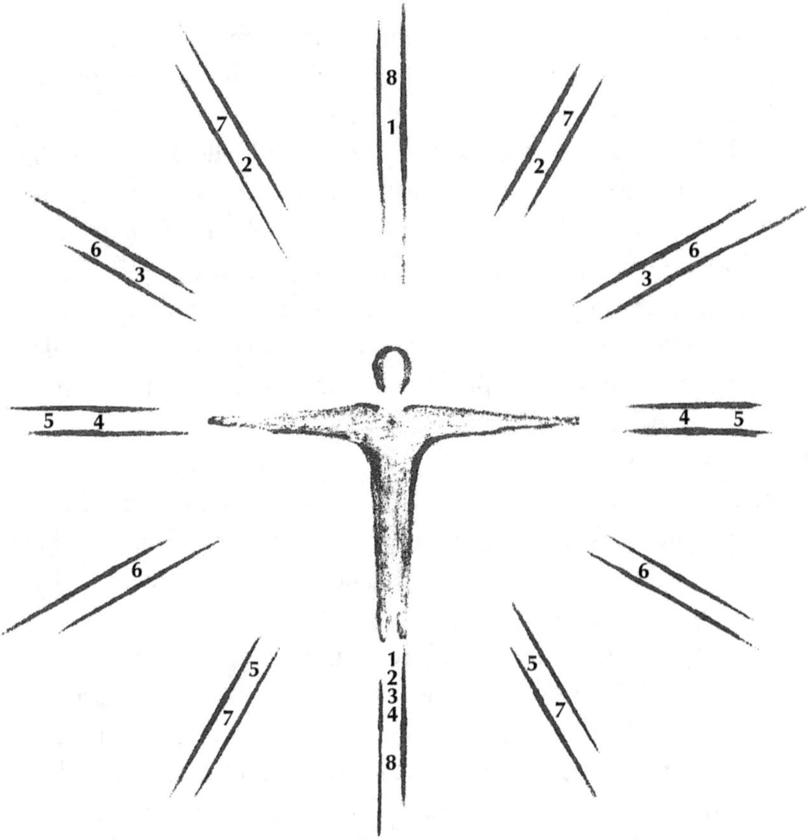

## 1. THE FIRST IMPULSE IN 1915

*The seven tones of the basic scale*
*(substituted from Zuccoli,* Aus der Toneurythmie-Arbeit*)*

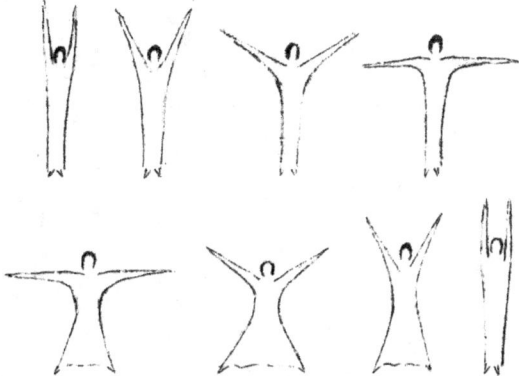

On August 23, 1915, Rudolf Steiner gave the very first indications for 'visible singing' – namely, the seven tones of the basic scale.

This first eurythmical archetypal scale of whole tones, with its exact mathematical angles that are related to the upright posture, divides the circumference into twelve equal segments of 30 degrees. Through the relationship of below and above – that is, through the way the angles of the arms and legs are related to each other in a differentiated manner – the scale brings to expression a picture of the laws of involution and evolution in the musical element.

The symmetry of right and left emphasises the element of feeling in which music lives. Each of these seven tone angles is a being unto itself and bears no relation to pitch. They are the expression for the soul-spiritual experience that is revealed by the sevenfoldness in the world.

Unfortunately, the archetype of the scale was too quickly grasped by the intellect. The musicians made the objection that the scale includes half tones. Rudolf Steiner immediately changed the degrees of the angle to correspond with J.S. Bach's well-tempered system. Seven years later, Rudolf Steiner pointed to the transformation of the seven whole tones into the scale we are familiar with today.[3]

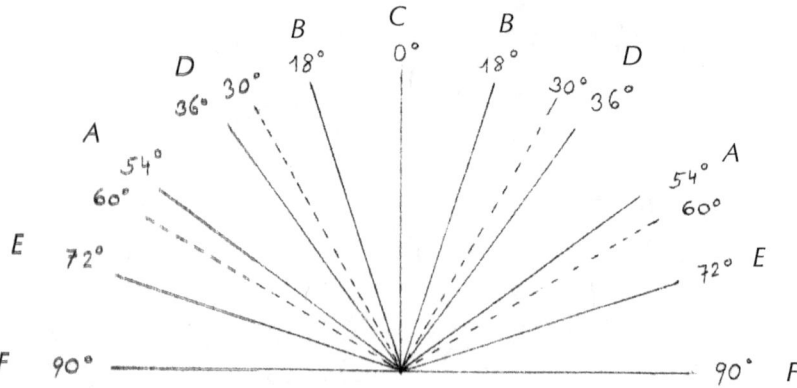

# 1. THE FIRST IMPULSE IN 1915

Looking at the movement of the first (lower) tetrachord, we have from the first to the fourth note a gesture that opens in its development until it becomes a cross on the fourth note. According to the law of sevenfoldness, a transformation takes place through a new impulse of will towards the second (upper) tetrachord. This is the striving towards the octave, the longing for a 'new birth in the spirit'. The duality of the first and second tetrachords is clearly experienced by practising eurythmists. It is also the basic principle for the future rhythmical forming of the intervals. Descending from the octave to the prime, we feel, in the movement of the upper tetrachord, as though we are taking leave of the gods. And in the movement from the fourth note to the prime, we feel as though what has been received by the gods is being enclosed in the centre of the heart.

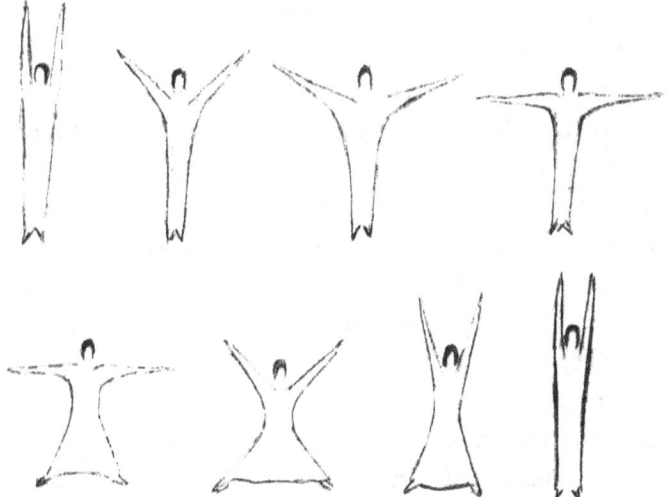

*Figures of the (major) scale*

Later on, through artistic practice, we paid attention to whether a tone or interval within a melody had an opening or closing character of movement.

The eurythmist Erna van Deventer asked whether these angles were tones or intervals, and Rudolf Steiner answered, 'In the long run you have to feel whether the movement is to be used for the note or for the interval.'[4]*

The lectures that Rudolf Steiner gave about music in 1915 help to develop a feeling for the nature and being of single tones. In lecture five of *Art as Seen in the Light of Mystery Wisdom,* he described how, in the future, human beings will experience the spiritual beingness of the tones. Today we only achieve this through meditative penetration into the tone. Rudolf Steiner urged us to hear the melody in the single tone.

In later lectures in Stuttgart and Dornach, he indicated how different the musical experience is for people today than it was in earlier cultural epochs. The difference lies in the change of consciousness and of the human constitution through the different Spirits of Time.[5]

Only today can major and minor be consciously grasped in our personal attitude of soul. Every tone can be experienced in major or minor – in the lightness of spirit or under the pressure of the weight of the earth. The urge in the human being to utter a tone is either an expression of the resistance against the danger of sinking into the depths or of a force that holds us back from wafting away into the world of light. This is an archetypal urge that seeks to create a balance in our soul through tone.

Rudolf Steiner therefore gave the angles in the minor scale below the shoulders as a mirror picture to the major scale. It is

---

* It is bewildering that the number seven contains both elements in the world: the *movement*, which develops through time, and the *condition*, which stays as it is. Therefore, the expression 'stage' is to be understood like the seven conditions of the earth evolution with Old Saturn, Old Sun, Old Moon, and so on, and, with the same designations, the planets and their movements. Both tone and interval live in time as 'pedal point' and as movement, which in the end will change into a fixed star and enter into duration.

# 1. THE FIRST IMPULSE IN 1915

palpable how differently the weight affects the arms depending on whether they are above or below the shoulders.

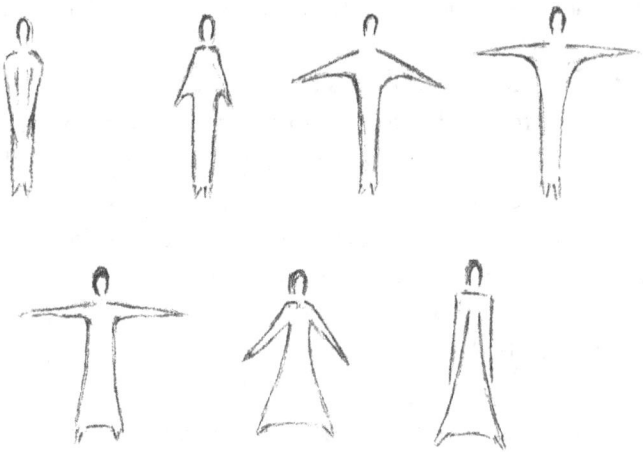

*Figures of the minor scale*

To the minor was added the fact that the hindering force of weight causes the angles of the arms and legs to be slightly compressed and thereby pushed a little forwards.

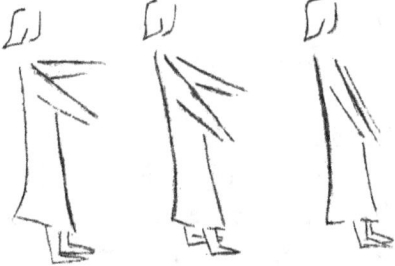

*Position of the body for the jumps in minor: G♭, A♭, B♭*

Many years later, despite the complicated forms in space, we still held strictly to 'above and below the shoulders' for major and minor because pitch was not yet taken into account. But that which can be experienced in the movement with regards to pressure and lightness should not be forgotten, even though many other indications, such as pitch or melos,* have been added.

Rudolf Steiner gave the possibility to do the angles in varied ways. For example, the degrees of the angles did not need to be done with the whole arm in relationship to the gestalt, to the spine, but could also be done in the elbow between upper and lower arm, in the wrist between hand and lower arm, or between thumb and fingers. In the sketch, the arrow on the dotted line is the place that is decisive for the experience of the angle. Obviously the angles of the legs remain the same for G, A, B, without any change.

That the angles of the tones only appear in the arms and hands – but nowhere else in the human gestalt – becomes clear through the lectures given nine years later.[6] The hands and arms – freed from the weight of earth through uprightness – belong to the middle rhythmical human being because they are connected to the collar bone (clavicle), which guides the streams that otherwise take hold of the larynx and directs them into the arms where visible singing arises. For this 'singing out', it is important that the stream is also perceived and that the movements of the angles radiate outwards, as shown in the sketch.

What Rudolf Steiner brought in the very first lessons has in no way been superseded by what followed or been made obsolete over the following years. This is confirmed, for instance, by the answer he gave nine years later, in the summer of 1924, when the eurythmist Friedel Thomas-Simons asked him how she should do quick tones in an arpeggio: 'Do the melos with the upper arm and the tones with the hands.'

---

* 'Melos' is a term that refers to the movement of the rising or falling of tones as opposed to the distinct degrees of highness or lowness of pitch. (*Translator*)

# 1. THE FIRST IMPULSE IN 1915

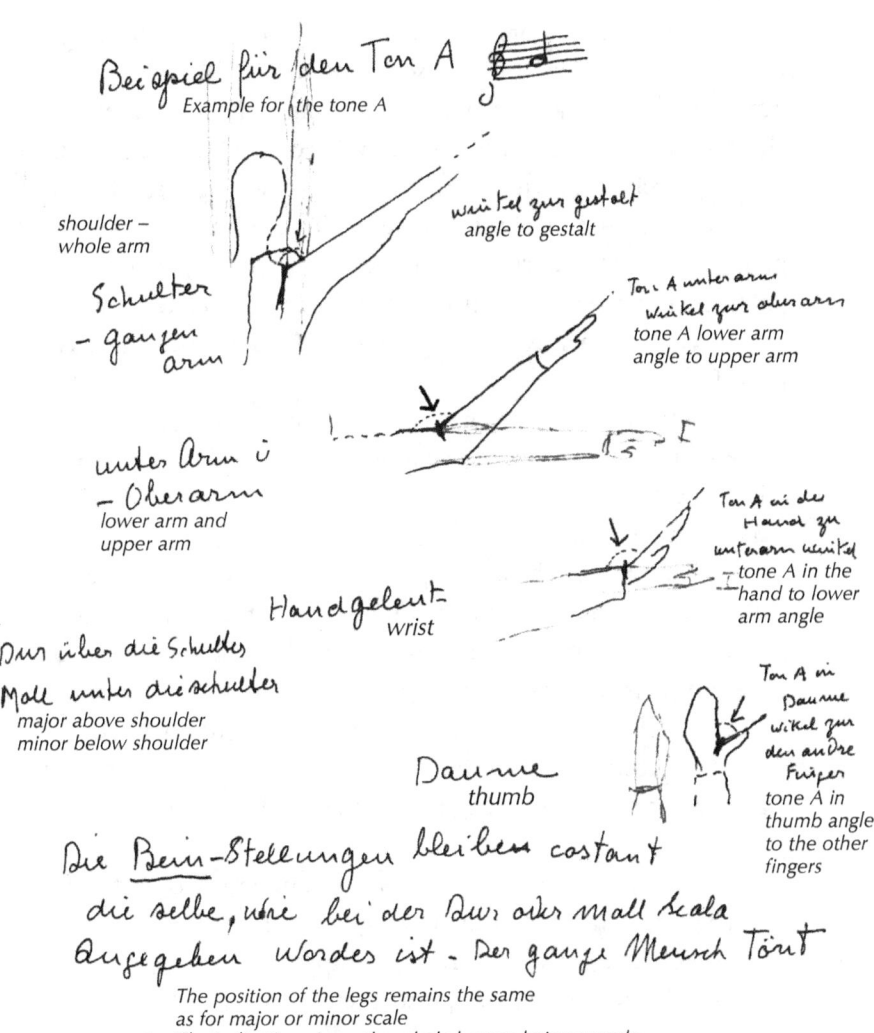

*Original sketch by Elena Zuccoli*

The movements of the angles, whether small or large, must be very exact, otherwise there will be a discrepancy between the physical arm movement and the movement of the etheric body. The etheric body follows what the human being perceives in the tone, speech sound, or mood, and does not follow the physical gesture. The physical eurythmy gesture must follow the etheric body; otherwise, there is no true experience of the gesture. Thus we can understand that a movement that arises out of conceptualisation does not have a spiritual reality.

In observing how speech and tone are differentiated in their movements, we can clearly see how we step out into the world with speech eurythmy, while, musically, we move in an inner world with the tones.

Thus we can understand that at the beginning of speech eurythmy, the movement was done in space (for instance, steps in alliteration) without arm gestures; and at the beginning of tone eurythmy, movements were done with the arms while standing. The difference between speech and tone eurythmy lies in the connection to the outer world in speech eurythmy and in the perception of the inner life in tone eurythmy.

> But then we really have to feel the connection between the world and the human being; we must feel how speech brings us into a relationship with the outer world, and music [tone] into a relationship with ourselves; how, in consequence, all the movements of speech eurythmy are, as it were, drawn from the human being and transplanted into the outer world, whereas the gestures of music[-eurythmy] have to flow back into the human being. Everything which goes out in speech-eurythmy has to lead back into the human being in music-eurythmy.[7]

This impulse of tone eurythmy was taken up and practised with great enthusiasm above all by Tatiana Kisseleff and Hendrika Hollenbach. It was wonderful to see how these two individuals dedicated themselves to this new impulse with such devotion.

It was an enormous task for the eurythmists in Dornach to put into practice the many new indications for speech eurythmy given in the course in 1915. This is evident from reports given by Marie Steiner and Tatiana Kisseleff.[8] This wealth of indications for speech eurythmy overshadowed the sparse indications of the seven tone angles. And Tatiana Kisseleff, who was the most experienced amongst the eurythmists, felt a responsibility towards the tone eurythmy indications and tried to practise the tones in her courses.

Soon, through the production of Goethe's *Faust*, she no longer had time to devote herself to this task. And so, it came about that Hollenbach, who was also a musician and pianist, took on the tone eurythmy and began to practise the angles of the tones with children in her music lessons. Only this work with children remained of the tone eurythmy impulse.


The First World War was still raging in Europe. For political reasons, many artists working on the Goetheanum building had to leave Switzerland. The war front was very close, and one could hear the thunder of artillery in Dornach. But the work on the building of the Goetheanum continued and demanded double the effort of those still present. Only Rudolf and Marie Steiner's extraordinary strength, devotion and sacrifices helped to overcome the difficulties that arose when people from warring nations lived and worked together. Rudolf and Marie Steiner were again and again able to awaken the consciousness that this work had cultural significance for the whole of humanity.

Marie Steiner took over the direction of the eurythmy rehearsals and at the same time developed the new art of speech formation – so absolutely essential for the life and existence of eurythmy.

When the war came to an end, it left an inner and outer disintegration. In many countries there was political unrest, revolutions broke out, and social structures disintegrated. In this chaos, Rudolf Steiner felt called upon to give Europe a new direction through the spiritual impulses of the threefold social order. Many social initiatives arose: the Waldorf School, biodynamic agriculture, the Christian Community, and much more.

Within the eurythmy work, new life also began. The very small artistic group in Dornach expanded and received new stimulus through Rudolf Steiner's standard forms, or 'Doctor Forms', as they were sometimes called.

Hendrika Hollenbach had further developed small tone eurythmy choruses with a group of children in Dornach. She showed her work to Marie Steiner, who was delighted. These children's choruses were taken up into the Sunday performances, received great applause, and inspired a few eurythmists to learn tone eurythmy. Hollenbach thereby had the opportunity to work on tone eurythmy with adults.

# 2

# Reawakened Interest in Tone Eurythmy

There was now a great surge of interest in tone eurythmy and there were regular practices on the stage in the Carpentry Shop. As Hendrika Hollenbach described:

> When Dr Steiner went through the Carpenters' Workshop there was an opportunity to ask questions. So we heard that we could certainly do notes whilst moving. In the major we now jumped for the notes G, A and B whilst moving, but how the different minor jumps could be indicated while moving was a problem. When I asked, Rudolf Steiner said that you have to restrain the movement. As I didn't immediately understand how he meant it, he let me do it. One step forward, then place the feet side by side, again a step, then feet together, and so on, so that in the sequence F, G, A, B, C, a strong slowing down, like a gentle hindrance comes out in the movement.[1]

To begin with, melodies and scales were practised with the type of stepping indicated for the tones G, A, and B of the upper tetrachord. But we soon discovered that, when the outer value of the note was very fast or slow, we could not coordinate the outer value of the notes with the iambic and trochaic steps that had been indicated for the upper tetrachord. Rudolf Steiner helped by giving different variations for the steps.

For the quick major tones G, A, and B, *both* feet move almost simultaneously. While the one leg jumps the short, the other leg does the long. Thus, a light, joyful skipping in iambic is the result (see sketch I).

For the long major tones for G, A, and B, he indicated that first the short, then the long – one after the other with the same foot – creates the iambic (see sketch II).

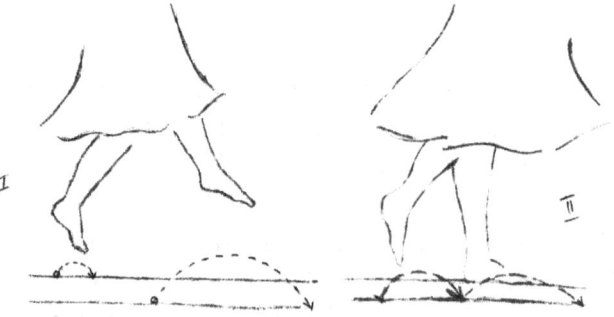

*Steps for quick major tones (I) and long major tones (II)*

In minor, G, A, and B long tones can be done with a normal trochee – that is, with both feet moving one after the other for a tone (no sketch for this); whereas with G, A, and B as quick

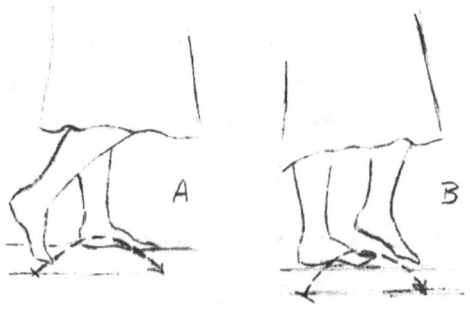

*Quick Minor Tone*
*A: starting with an open step.*     *B: starting with feet together*

# 2. REAWAKENED INTEREST IN TONE EURYTHMY

minor tones, the step for the trochee changes into only a half-step with *one* foot.

With minor, we should make sure that, at the end of the trochee for G, A, and B, the weight in minor becomes visible through the experience of pressure; thus, the eurythmist takes on the same position as the one for the minor tones in standing (see page 21).

In order to be performed, these major and minor steps now needed forms in space. Rudolf Steiner gave straight lines for major and round forms for minor, neither of which was bound to any specific spatial direction.

Hendrika Hollenbach received a tone spiral form from Rudolf Steiner that was quite different from the one given to Kisseleff in 1915. This tone spiral encompasses five octaves, corresponding to the range of tones within the human experience. The numbers twelve, seven, five, three, and one are contained in this spiral: there are twelve radii, seven tones of the scale, the triads that appear on each radius, and the single tone as such. The bass notes are in the centre of the spiral and the high tones are on the periphery. Here a rhythmic, geometric relationship between the voices comes to expression in the pitch.

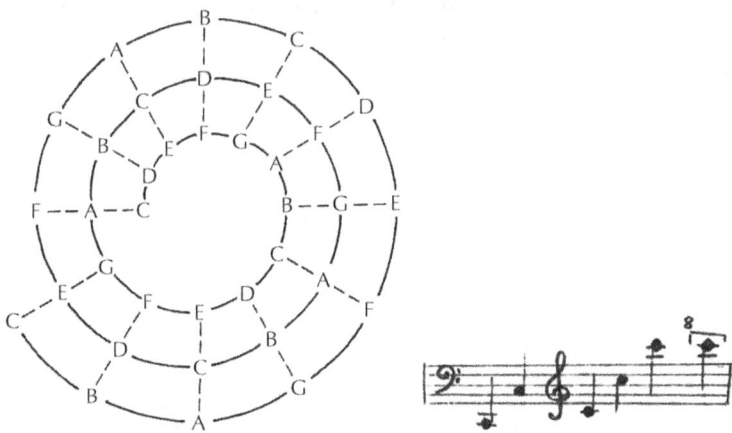

At that time, eurythmy was part of personal schooling. Many members practised daily on their own. It was a heartfelt wish to experience anthroposophy not only through strict thinking but also through art.

This inner religious feeling that every artist must have – for art can only be grasped through feeling – was powerfully alive and stimulated by Rudolf Steiner's presence. The performances of the small stage group at the Goetheanum (the only existing one), which was under the directorship of Rudolf Steiner himself, had reached such a high level that the solemn mood of celebration had a powerful effect on the audience. The humoresques were filled with such brilliant wit that one had to laugh out of the depths of the heart. Nevertheless, they did not lose their impact of leading to healthy self-knowledge.

In the artistic work, both in speech and tone eurythmy, we always tried to bring out the inherent characteristic qualities through eurythmy. For this was what Rudolf Steiner wanted to see, and he nearly always helped us to find it. It was striking how this could be brought out by him through the simplest eurythmical means.

Tone eurythmy developed significantly through the fact that Rudolf Steiner created tone eurythmy forms. From 1922 onwards, the programmes included the most beautiful tone pieces.

# 3

# The Birth of the First Eurythmy School

In the autumn of 1922, there was a turning point in the development of eurythmy. Inner and outer factors demanded decisive measures. Groups and anthroposophical institutions that arose in many areas all wanted eurythmy for their work.

Marie Steiner, who was responsible for the development of eurythmy, saw the necessity of establishing a training centre. Rudolf Steiner supported her in this, and helped to bring it about. They decided on Stuttgart for the training, where Waldorf teachers were trained who were able to teach the supporting subjects.

In October 1922 a first class commenced as a trial. Rudolf Steiner gave the leadership of the school to Alice Fels who had taken part in everything anthroposophical for years and had acquired a thorough knowledge of eurythmy. The responsibility for tone eurythmy was given to Hedwig Köhler who was also a musician and had worked as a eurythmist in the stage group in Dornach. She was someone who had a rich imagination and was entirely different in every way from Alice Fels. Rudolf Steiner expected the subject teachers to work with their subject matter in a way that was fruitful for the eurythmy students. The class consisted of a very cosmopolitan group of students.

For the time being, the Eurythmy School was located in the house of the Anthroposophical Society. There was a beautiful stage, which, like everything else in the hall, was painted a dark indigo blue. The only decorations were the large, golden planetary seals carved into the blue wood. Classes began at seven o'clock in the morning and the seminars took place in the evenings. Erich Schwebsch, an enthusiastic admirer of Anton Bruckner, taught music.

Rudolf Steiner came to Stuttgart almost every week, and because his lodgings were in the same house, he looked in on the lessons as often as he could, giving advice and suggestions. He encouraged the school to have the eurythmy students perform every month. This had various effects. For instance, the Stuttgart members of the Anthroposophical Society, who at first looked somewhat sceptically on the new art school, gradually developed a different attitude. The eurythmy teachers required strict self-knowledge, a constant stimulus to their powers of imagination, and no room for laziness in the lessons. The students had to stay awake and be diligent in order to keep up with the demands of the training. All that was performed at that time made a deep impression in the memory of those present.

After returning from the winter holidays in January 1923, deeply shaken by the news of the burning of the first Goetheanum on New Year's Eve, everyone took hold of the work with renewed strength of will.

Hedwig Köhler, inspired by the lectures of Erich Schwebsch, began boldly working with the students on a movement from Bruckner's *Eighth Symphony*. This was a huge project, as the students had only studied tone eurythmy for one term. Everyone did their best. They attempted to do this symphony in eurythmy on a podium with three levels. It required a great deal of technical skill to remain facing the front while climbing up and down. Köhler tried to bring to expression the character of the instruments through specific movements of the arms. Schwebsch often stood by her side and offered musical advice. The aim was to show the work to Rudolf Steiner in March when his lectures on music would take place.

In addition to the Waldorf teachers, eurythmists were also allowed to attend these lectures on music because, as well as giving the basis for music lessons, he gave many impulses for the artistic element, as well as for an understanding of the situation of music in our times. In the two lectures, Rudolf Steiner showed how fruitful and stimulating education can be if it seeks to understand life by considering the human being and the world in connection with one another. These lectures are models for a method of teaching by which we can arrive at the essential.[1]

The evolution of the earth as a musical process can be experienced anew through the description of how human consciousness has changed throughout the cultural epochs in connection to the seven tones. We come to recognise what people of today can grasp through the world of tones. Since the appearance of the musical interval of the fourth, human beings feel themselves as self-contained beings, as microcosms. By grasping their own self, they find in inner seclusion the joy and sorrow that are revealed as the experience of major and minor within the nature of the third.

If this is grasped through a musical feeling in the rhythm of the heart and lungs, then it is experienced as *harmony;* when the musical element extends to the head, it is experienced as *melody;* through the circulation of the blood the musical experience in the limbs becomes *rhythm*. (This explains why Rudolf Steiner gave us the rhythmical forms of the seven intervals for eurythmy as they express themselves as rhythmical movements in our will.)

Thus, the musical human being becomes visible in cosmic form, which also appears in the harmonious sounding of an orchestra. In the harmony, rhythm and melos of symphonic works the cosmic image appears of how the feeling, willing and thinking human being of the spheres is revealed in the cosmos in the form of song.

In speech eurythmy, the soul forces of thinking, feeling, and willing is an expression of the *whole* human being – head, chest, and limbs. In tone eurythmy, the middle part is active – heart and lungs. This part only partially grasps the head and limbs. Therefore, in tone eurythmy, one cannot speak of thinking, feeling, and willing, but rather of how feeling in the head becomes melos, and feeling in the will expresses itself as rhythm. The heart perceives the harmony of the tones.

> The centre of music today is harmony ... The element of harmony takes hold directly of human feeling. What is expressed in harmonies is experienced by human feeling ... In looking at the human being, we can say that we have feeling in the middle ...
>
> ... One thus can say that while the melody is carried from the heart to the head on the stream of breath ... the rhythm is carried on the waves of the blood circulation from the heart to the limbs, and in the limbs it is arrested as willing. From this you can see how the musical element really pervades the whole human being.
>
> Picture the whole human being who experiences the musical element as a human spirit: the ability to experience the element of melody gives you the head of this spirit. The ability to experience the element of harmony gives you the chest, the central organ of this spirit; and the ability to experience the rhythm gives

you the limbs of this spirit. What have I described for you here? I have described the human etheric body. If only you depict the whole musical experience, and if you do this correctly, you actually have before you the human etheric body. It is just that instead of 'head' we say, 'melody'; instead of 'rhythmic man' – because it is lifted upward – we say 'harmony'; and instead of 'limb man' – we cannot say here, 'metabolic man' – we say, 'rhythm'. We have the entire human being etherically before us.[2]

Immediately after the lectures, all the new indications were practised diligently and shown to Rudolf Steiner in order to receive the invaluable corrections that, unfortunately, were often not written down.

Firstly, Steiner was shown the gesture for the octave, which Köhler had tried with us as a two-tone chord with Chopin's *Prelude in C minor,* Op. 28, No. 20. This movement consisted in simultaneously forming the two tones of the octave in mirror image up and down. With this, only the pitch of the two tones was taken into consideration, and the gesture was a long way from what Rudolf Steiner gave later as the gesture for the interval of the octave. Melos was still unknown.

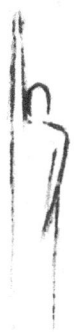

*Gesture for the octave*

Not only was the Prelude done with arm gestures, but the round and straight forms were added according to major and minor, as well as the corresponding rhythms of the major and minor tones in the feet. It was truly majestic.

What had thus far differentiated the first (lower) and second (upper) tetrachord in a general way now became modified with rhythmical, wilful curves – backward for the first tetrachord and forward for the second. (The forms are always drawn from the audience's point of view.)

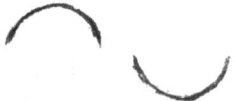

To remain musical, the curves must be done with a feeling for how the movement differs inwardly, depending on whether the curve is done forward or backward. Here it is not a matter of forms that enter into space.*

> If you focus on what is said here, you will grasp better the forms that appear in our tone eurythmy. You will also grasp something else. You will, for example, grasp the reason that out of instinct the feeling will arise to interpret the lower segments of the octave – the prime, second, and third – by backward movements and in the case of the upper tones – the fifth, sixth, and seventh – by forward movements.[3]

We find these curves of the lower and upper tetrachords applied in the tone eurythmy forms given by Rudolf Steiner.

Through the detailed and colourful description of the individual intervals of the scale, the feeling arose that a

---

* See Steiner's notes for *Eurythmy as Visible Singing* (p. 197): 'In the *musical element* the spatial human being is transformed into the non-spatial human being – the spiritual human being is the *inner* origin of the musical element.' *(Translator)*

# 3. THE BIRTH OF THE FIRST EURYTHMY SCHOOL

differentiated will-impulse that has its own expression lives in every tone.* In order to make the spiritual differentiation of the upper tones of the scale even more visible, Rudolf Steiner gave to the curves of the upper tetrachord the character of each of these intervals. He established the possibility for the differentiation of the fifth, sixth, and seventh.

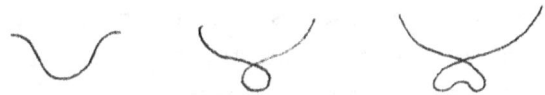

> The interval of the fifth is a real experience of imagination. He who can experience fifths correctly is actually in a position to know on the subjective level what imagination is like. One who experiences sixths knows what inspiration is. Finally, one who fully experiences sevenths – if he survives this experience – knows what intuition is. What I mean is that in the experience of the seventh the form of the soul's composition is the same as clairvoyantly with intuition. The form of the soul's composition during the experience of the sixth is that of inspiration with clairvoyance. The experience of the fifth is a real imaginative experience.[4]

---

* The inner rhythm of the individual tone: 1. standing, 2. stepping major, 3. stepping minor, 4. rhythmical forms.

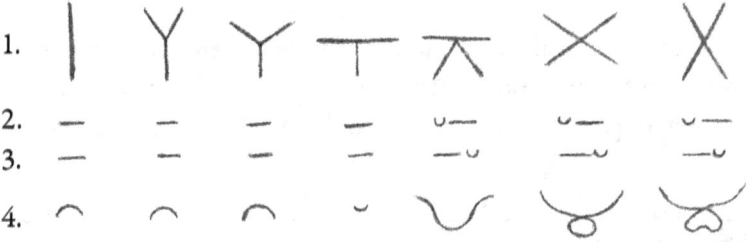

Rudolf Steiner drew these rhythmical forms on the blackboard. As no one dared to erase them, they remained there a long time, and one could look at these forms every day. They were diligently practised, also in their possible variations – with major, they were somewhat straighter, with minor, somewhat rounder; for the very high tones, the fingers were more pointed, while for lower ones, they were rounder.

As these rhythmical forms were not drawn on black paper, as was the custom then, unfortunately, we do not have the originals anymore.* The forms were passed on, in some cases incorrectly.

For the pure interval of the fourth, he asked for a movement that is held back, and thus he drew the form for the fourth with only a very short line.

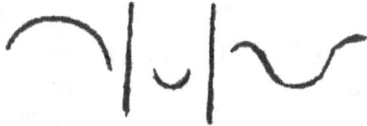

The human beings really experience hemselves as etheric body in the experience of the fourth, but a kind of summation forms within them. The experience of the fourth contains a touch of melody, a touch of harmony, a touch of rhythm, but all interwoven in such a way that they are no longer distinguishable. The entire human being is experienced spiritually at the threshold in the experience of the fourth: one experiences the etheric human being.[5]

Great technical control was demanded by the three different movements for melos, harmony and rhythm because Rudolf Steiner requested very precise angles at the same time as the

---

* Now that we can see Rudolf Steiner's drawings in his notebook, we can see that Elena Zuccoli's drawings are as close to the original as possible. [*Translator*]

# 3. THE BIRTH OF THE FIRST EURYTHMY SCHOOL

rhythmical interval forms and the harmony of major and minor. When achieved, this was impressively beautiful: the spirit-soul nature differentiated musically in the human being could be experienced directly, and, at the same time, melos, harmony and rhythm became a unity.

The Bruckner Symphony was shown to Rudolf Steiner. Whenever a new initiative arose, he was able to introduce new things and present unexpected points of view and possibilities – in this instance, the possibilities that lie hidden in the art of tone eurythmy.

Surprisingly, and quite unexpectedly, Rudolf Steiner rejected any attempt to characterise the various instruments through the movements of the arms. He clearly indicated that in tone eurythmy the arms are to be moved exclusively for visible singing. But the *forms in space,* on the other hand, should be carried out so that the characteristic form of the instrument appears.*

Rudolf Steiner had a large podium placed in the middle of the stage and a smaller one on top. On the smaller podium, as the central and highest point, stood the timpani; on the larger one below stood all the other percussion instruments.

The brass instruments were to move radially between the centre and the periphery.

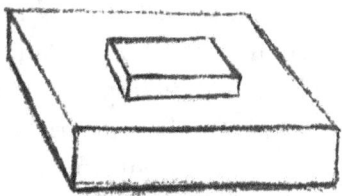

The strings, whose form-principle is the lemniscate, encircle the whole in many variations – slimmer or thicker according to the instrument.

---

* Rudolf Steiner's well-known indication, 'pointed fingers for the flute,' applies only to the character of the piece (Minuet for Flute and Piano after a Song by William Rosenberg) and not for the flute generally.

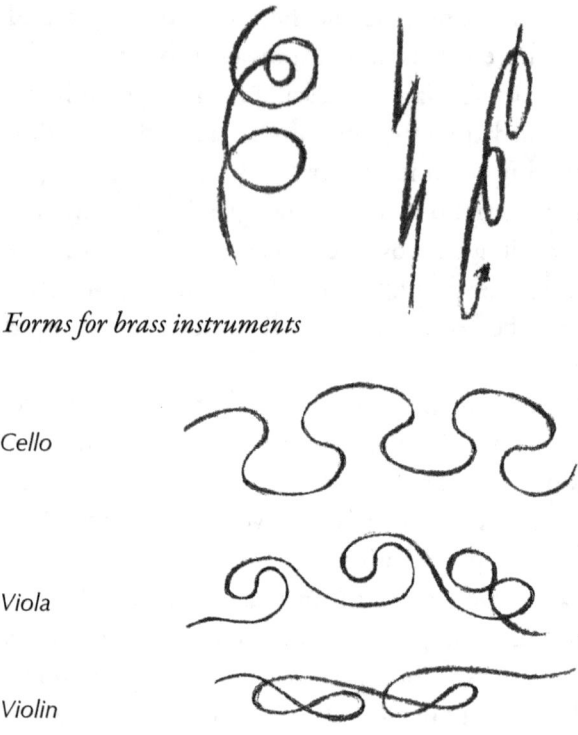

*Forms for brass instruments*

Cello

Viola

Violin

*Forms for string instruments*

The orchestra is a unity, an image of the *cosmic* human being of will (percussive instruments standing in the middle), of feeling (strings encircling the podium), and of the thinking element (wind instruments radiating from the centre to the periphery). Köhler drew new forms corresponding to these indications, and soon the symphonic movement could appear in its second form with a thoroughly cosmic dimension.

When it was ready, the students were allowed to show it to Rudolf Steiner in this symphonic archetype (which lies hidden in every orchestral piece) in order to receive further indications. Now it was possible, for the first time, to progress from the archetype to an artistic presentation. He gave the difficult task of 'folding over' the entire circular movement to arrive at a

# 3. THE BIRTH OF THE FIRST EURYTHMY SCHOOL

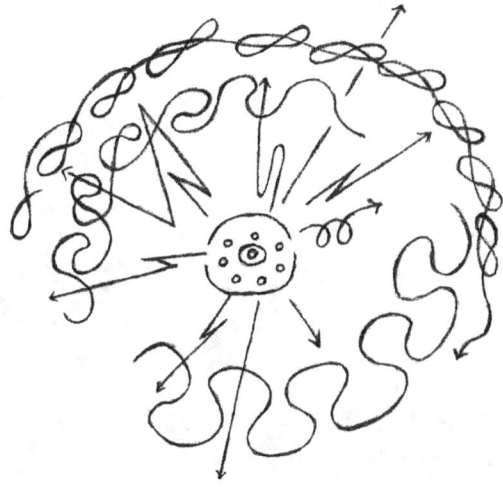

form appropriate to the stage. The percussion instruments had to move to the back, and the whole was adapted to a semicircle and rehearsed anew for a third time. This was much more difficult to arrange because the harmonies were supposed to appear through the relationship of the instruments to each other. Many new problems arose, and although there was a timid attempt to solve them at the time, there are still questions to this day. By summer, the whole symphony was finished at last and was performed for the public.

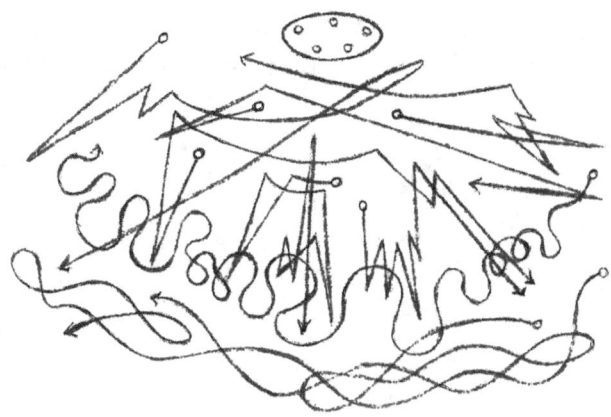

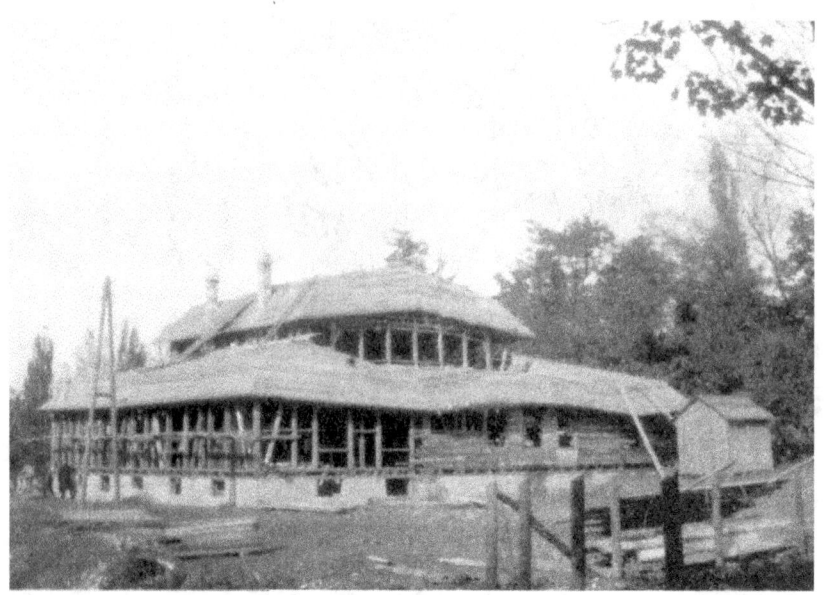

*The First Eurythmy School in Stuttgart (during construction), by permission of Ingrid Braunschmidt*

In 1923, many new students were accepted, for there was a great wish to study eurythmy. Due to a shortage of rooms, the eurythmy students had to practise in the Waldorf School before classes began. But this meant that the first practice sessions had to begin at six o'clock in the morning. During the winter months this was quite an imposition. The decision was then taken to build a eurythmy school as soon as possible.

4

# The Christmas Conference 1923/24

The Eurythmy School was invited to the new founding of the Anthroposophical Society in Dornach. The school was to participate in this event by giving a performance during the conference.

In Dornach, a blanket of snow covered the ground as the conference participants arrived on December 23, 1923. At the entrances to the Goetheanum grounds stood watchmen, wearing thick fur coats and hats. They guarded the whole area and did not allow unauthorised entry. Seen from Haus de Jaager, they looked enormous against the evening sky. Most of them were artists who had worked over the years on the building. They now had the task to conscientiously safeguard Rudolf Steiner's life and to protect the sculpture and the whole site around the Goetheanum.

The dress rehearsal for the Stuttgart students took place during the conference. In the audience there were many members from Dornach, as well as eurythmists and musicians from the Goetheanum. Rudolf Steiner was also present, as he was at every eurythmy dress rehearsal. The programme included a short song for voice and piano by Jean Sibelius. Köhler, who had been a singer, sang for the eurythmy. Suddenly, Rudolf Steiner interrupted the rehearsal, and, turning to the musicians, he angrily asked: 'How can one do something so inartistic – tone eurythmy with singing?' The musicians were especially taken aback by this statement. Had not Jan Stuten from time to time sung a song by Bach for eurythmy? But Rudolf Steiner must have felt that he needed to interfere radically, and he cancelled the whole programme because of these few measures of artistic error.*

A new programme was quickly organised with the Dornach eurythmists. Only two solos – Maria Jenny-Schuster and Elena Zuccoli – and a few group pieces were included in the Dornach conference programme by Marie Steiner.

This strict reaction was puzzling for quite a few people because it was not clear what Rudolf Steiner had meant, and his admonition had an effect like none other. None of those affected were sad or even angry that the whole autumn's work was not included. The immensely spiritual, elevated mood of the Christmas Conference did not allow for any personal rancour to arise. We were present at such a great spiritual event that all mundane concerns disappeared.

In retrospect, during these Christmas days, it was as if we had been transported to a high mountaintop and lived far above the surrounding world.

---

* Although Rudolf Steiner gave a few indications concerning the problem of singing and tone eurythmy movement in his introductory words before the eurythmy performance at the conference, it was only during the Tone Eurythmy Course shortly afterwards in February 1924 (*Eurythmy as Visible Singing*) that it was possible to understand where the error lay. Seventy years later the problem arose again with various experiments. But they all led to the same conclusion, that the eurythmy gestures, both for speech and tone, are not yet differentiated enough in their basic, individual character. That remains true up to the present.

# 5

# New Foundations of Tone Eurythmy

## February 1924

Nine years after the beginning of tone eurythmy, the urgently needed Tone Eurythmy Course took place. The tone eurythmy impulses of 1915 and 1924 are attempts by Rudolf Steiner to awaken the musical element in the human being in different ways.

The Therapeutic Course (*Eurythmy Therapy*) was given to medical doctors in 1921. It was instigated by two eurythmists, Elisabeth Baumann-Dollfus and Erna van Deventer-Wolfram.

In 1924, there was still a great discrepancy between the development of speech and of tone eurythmy. In the first years, eurythmists gained significant experience regarding the possibilities of movement in speech eurythmy through the production of *Faust,* which fructified the imagination and developed their skills.

Although Rudolf Steiner had also recently created forms for tone eurythmy, the dearth of gestures in contrast to the perfection of the given forms was remarkable. That is why he opened the course with the words: 'And this is also why I believe it to be necessary that now we should at least *begin* to lay down the foundation of [tone] music-eurythmy.'[1]

The first and only foundational tone course has its own character. It took place in the eurythmy room of the Glass House. The mood was intimate, as we were still full of impressions from the Christmas Conference.

Most of the participants were people who had lived in Dornach for years and were familiar with the concepts of spiritual science. He therefore only needed to give brief allusions to call to mind what we already knew – for example, the lectures about the human senses (*A Psychology of Body, Soul, and Spirit*), which Steiner gave in October of 1909 to help seeking artists of that time.

The whole course is an example of how the Goethean method can be put into practice in art. If we survey the development of the eight lectures of the course, we can feel it as a scale from the prime to the octave and can also use it as an ideal structure for teaching tone eurythmy. The artists find in the given sequence of eurythmical laws a support for their powers of imagination, as well as ample stimulation for artistic creative possibilities.

Just as musicians must come to know their instrument thoroughly in all its parts, its form and its substance, in order to master it, so Rudolf Steiner showed the eurythmists how the human spirit and soul can master the body as an instrument.

What we already knew about eurythmy at that time was only briefly mentioned. Everything in the course was completely new for us.

Rudolf Steiner began the course at the boundary where speech and tone diverge:

> Speech is the relationship of the human being to the world. Music is the relationship of the human being, as a being of soul and spirit, to him- or herself.[2]

## 5. NEW FOUNDATIONS OF TONE EURYTHMY

The longer one lives with the first lecture, the more one learns to understand its comprehensive content and the foundational indications for the prerequisites of an art of eurythmy. Here Rudolf Steiner demonstrated the character of all the eurythmy exercises, both for the artist and for the eurythmist in training.

The first condition is to know world evolution in the sense of Rudolf Steiner's anthroposophy, and thus to feel what the 'word' in the human being means.

With the first tone eurythmy movement, Rudolf Steiner challenged us to feel the difference in our gestalt between the direction-giving quality of the head and the movement of the feet. This established, in advance, the relationship of the octave to the prime; at the same time it awakened the possibility of gradually learning to perceive how the life force, which streams through the gestalt, can be grasped in the inner process of movement. We had received the indication in which the movement of the head forwards or backwards determines the step – either into the light world of major or the darkened, hindering world of minor. The arms, released from gravity, are then able to follow the soul-weaving of the intimate, mobile third, which, together with the formative force of the fifth, unites with the step of the prime. In this way, the basic musical chord in the human being is formed as an image of the cosmic trinity of the heights of the starry heavens, the sun's encircling widths and the earth depths.

To reawaken the lost sense for the musical, Rudolf Steiner emphasised the connections between music and speech. He began directly with the vowel A (*ah*), the alpha- or aleph-being that has been active in the human constitution throughout the ages and seeks to unite within the human being all the possibilities of movement that exist in the world.

Only in the fifth cultural epoch did there slowly awaken the consciousness for the interval of the third and thereby the possibility for human beings to experience major and minor. Thus, the feeling can arise in us that we are beings who live in two worlds. In language, this polarity between major and minor appears in the vowels A (*ah*) and E (as in g*a*te) within the element of minor, and O (*oh*) and U (*oo*) within the element of major. That element in us which produces and drives everything musical, and which also calls forth our soul-spiritual balance, remains mysteriously hidden. This is the individual, personal force of the I (*ee*) sound, which is the 'I' in the human being. To awaken this experience of the I (*ee*) sound, Rudolf Steiner gives the I-A-O head-exercise from back to front, and from front to back, so that the difference of these three sounds can be experienced.

Rudolf Steiner's many indications given before he came to the concluding movement of the triad are often not sufficiently observed, both in teaching and in personal practice. They consist of many suggestions that are very helpful but are easily overlooked by the intellect, which considers them 'already known'. They expand the experience of the realm of major and minor to include a broader range of differentiated sensations. This is true both for the inner feelings in life and for the outer forms of the various tensions and relaxations of one's own muscles, which are familiar through experiences of the conditions of soul and body in life. How different are the effects for the bodily feeling if a person is sanguine or melancholic; how different, for instance, is major and minor with a phlegmatic Roman like Corelli, or a fighter for the spirit like Beethoven. And how different is a human being's attitude of soul in health or illness.

Thus, we learn from the very beginning to be aware of our inner perceptions so that we can master the differentiated starting point of a single gesture. The audience perceives the inner mood in the *starting point* of the movement and not in the outer gesture of the eurythmist.

## 5. NEW FOUNDATIONS OF TONE EURYTHMY

Air and warmth are the bearers of the astral element and the 'I' in the human being. What the ear hears as sense organ is only the shadow of the tone in the element of the air. Rudolf Steiner describes the birth of the eurythmy gesture in his notes with the following sparse words:

> The *musical sound* and the *sound of speech:* they are occurrences in the astral body (air) and ego (warmth) – whereby the soul goes into itself – and forms the *gesture* reproducing the reflection in the physical body ... With the gesture the feeling (central) is the observer.[3]

Because we can only grasp music with our feeling, it is necessary, first of all, to develop our feeling into an organ capable of grasping the experience of major and minor. Major and minor give the impulse to all expressions of sound because major and minor attest to the freedom or limitation of the human soul.

Rudolf Steiner then leads us to the more intimate perception of the spirit-soul processes in the comprehensive sevenfoldness of the intervals. Here we encounter an obstacle that needs to be overcome.

> What otherwise remains an experience of the ear or larynx only, now has to become an experience of the whole human being. When it becomes an experience of the whole human being, it quite naturally becomes gesture. Once the experience is understood, is laid hold of, then the experience becomes gesture.[4]

The seven intervals are intimate, inaudible experiences, graspable in the stream of time between two sense-perceptible, audible tones. Over the years, much confusion has arisen, and many essential aspects have been lost. In the early days, the interval gestures were done with only one arm. But soon Rudolf Steiner made the remark that it was possible to do the gestures with both arms and that *only the seventh* should be done exclusively with *one* arm. When necessary, the other arm could, *without stretching,* join in the same direction as the stretched arm as a gentle accompaniment.

The *prime* lives hidden in the will. There is no hand or arm movement, and the prime step is only an indication of major or minor, depending on the musical context.

Just as in 1915 the original *second* was formed in the angle of the tone through a movement opening from C to D, so now the closed hand opens in a mood of expectation, with the palm horizontal, facing upwards in a questioning gesture.

Then comes the *third* with the up and down movement of the hand, demonstrated by Rudolf Steiner, which is an expression of the human as a being enclosed within itself.

Out of the open hand the finger tips in the *fourth* are drawn together, and, in rounding, create a space or an image of how the soul is enveloped in its etheric body before birth.

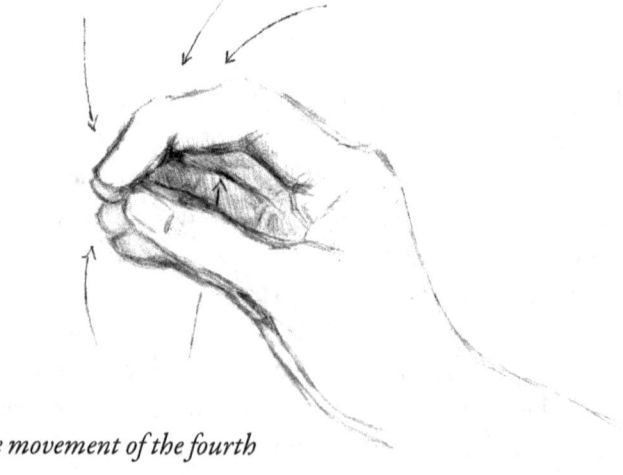

*The movement of the fourth*

## 5. NEW FOUNDATIONS OF TONE EURYTHMY

The feeling of the inner hand is led onto the back of the hand and, through the added movement of the arm, the gesture gains a formative force which belongs to the *fifth*. Here also, we can refer back to the transformation of the angle of the tone for the fourth (tone F), whose position on the cross (of the vertical body and the horizontal arms) becomes a fifth through a jump.

The movement of the *sixth* is given by Rudolf Steiner as a moving forward of the whole gestalt in the direction of the arm movements, which tells us that cosmic feeling and human feeling, in both directions, are interweaving and permeating each other. That is why the gesture of the interval of the sixth remains unchanged, be it ascending or descending. It is in balance between the cosmic spirit and the human soul at the same time. This is an archetype for the art of eurythmy in the far distant future.

> When we try to lower the life-spirit into the spirit-self, we will have to be living entirely in an element which as yet is absolutely strange to us. So what we can say in this domain is like the babbling of an infant before it has learnt to speak properly.[5]

In contrast to the sixth, the movement of the *seventh* is a losing of oneself through the out-streaming of life in order to reach the octave. The vibration of the hand and fingers arises out of the tension of striving to reach it.

If the seventh does *not* reach the octave, the hand stiffens, becomes lifeless in space. The gestalt comes to its aid, steps towards the lifeless, rigid hand and streams life back through the hand and arm towards the prime. The human being gains new life forces.

Rudolf Steiner showed the gesture for the *octave*, as recorded in the shorthand note, with the hand facing outwards and then turning towards oneself. The octave becomes the new prime.

> In the transition from keynote to octave, the octave simply falls into the keynote. It is as if you stretched out your hand and came into contact with an object. Through this external touch the longing you felt for something outside yourself is satisfied.[6]

Just as one can clearly see in the angles of the scale, and in the rhythmical interval forms, a differentiation of the movement for the first and second tetrachords, so, too, is this differentiation recognisable in the gestures of the intervals. With the first tetrachord, which is bound to the bodily-soul organism, the interval movements are mainly in the hands. In the second tetrachord, where the tones work on the spirit-soul organisation, the movements of the arms and the gestalt are added.

The gestures that were given are the conditions for the existence of the intervals. But each time, they must be formed by the artist in a way that is suited to the character of the motif without losing their essential qualities.

For present-day consciousness, the intervals of the prime, second and octave, in spite of their audible sounds, are not yet grasped spiritually. But they are nevertheless active, both in the physical as well as the soul-spiritual human constitution.

In order to achieve mobility in soul life and outer skill in the limbs, Rudolf Steiner gave eurythmy exercises for the intervals of the prime, third, fifth, and seventh in various sequences. These eurythmical movements of the intervals are spiritual-soul gestures that, as a spiritual researcher, he conveyed to us out of the imaginative world; they bear life within them. That is why it is necessary that they be practised *correctly,* even in their purely outward aspect. But they must be complemented by other exercises that lead to the inner experience in hearing.

## 5. NEW FOUNDATIONS OF TONE EURYTHMY

> Try first of all to become inwardly completely quiet, indifferent to sense impressions, as well as to any inward passion. Having achieved this state of indifference, sit down at the piano and play one of the middle notes – any note will do – and try while going up the scale to the octave really to experience the progression of notes.
>
> Having experienced this in peace and quiet, stand up and try to realise in eurythmy gestures what you have experienced. You will arrive at much, both in regard to what I have already mentioned and to those things about which I have still to speak. Endeavour, when attempting to reproduce in gesture what you have just played (single notes in an ascending progression) to bring into the eurythmy gestures (into the gestures for the triad, for instance) something similar to the gestures we have been discussing during these last few days. You will find it comparatively easy to feel a very strong connection between what you produce, feel and experience as gesture, and the notes as you play them successively on the piano.[7]

Through the two exercises, the outer gestures and the inner experience in hearing gradually come closer to each other until they become a unity. Then eurythmy is free to create art.

At the beginning of the course, Rudolf Steiner presented the human gestalt in its uprightness as the image of the cosmic trinity of height, depth, and widths. He then guided us to the experience of time through the seven eurythmy gestures of the musical intervals, which reveal in the soul the sevenfold nature of the life of the 'I' – a mirror of the laws of the seven stages of evolution.

Now he led us further, allowing us to grasp how the human skeleton is an imprint of the cosmic trinity of *melos, rhythm* and *beat,* which have been active throughout the ages and have fashioned the form of the body out of the depths of the earth.

If we look at the arrangement and forms of the bones, we see clearly the different characters of the three dimensions as images of the astral, etheric, and physical bodies. These find expression eurythmically in the stream of time through melos, rhythm and beat.

In the vertical, the forms of the bones are wonderfully ordered according to the laws of metamorphosis, an image of the forces of the astral body that is active in *melos*.

If we direct our attention to the difference between front and back in the forms of the bones, a completely different world is revealed. The forms show the contrast between the surfaces of the backs of the bones, which are closed off and create a boundary with the outer world, and the forms of the front of the bones that are open and receptive to the world. These qualities extend through the whole organism, even to the skin. For instance, consider how different our experience is of the inside of the hand in contrast to the outside. We perceive completely different degrees of sensitvity, as stark as the change in human life between waking and sleeping, day and night. It is the etheric body that is active here in different degrees, as a being of light, expressing itself in *rhythm*. Here, we live with the cosmic widths.

If we look at the human gestalt from the front, we will notice the symmetrical order of the bones. The differentiated forces of weight live invisibly here, where the will acts either more outwardly or more inwardly – two worlds, expressed as right and left in the musical-eurythmical *beat*.

*Melos* was done eurythmically in various ways. The essential aspect is that the movement follows the transformation of the tone upwards or downwards. Here, Rudolf Steiner gave

## 5. NEW FOUNDATIONS OF TONE EURYTHMY

a gesture in which we can most intensely experience the movement of the astral body. It consists in following the rising tone with the hand turned outwards, pointing upwards with the fingers, and following the falling tone with the flattened hand turned downwards, experiencing pressure or weight.

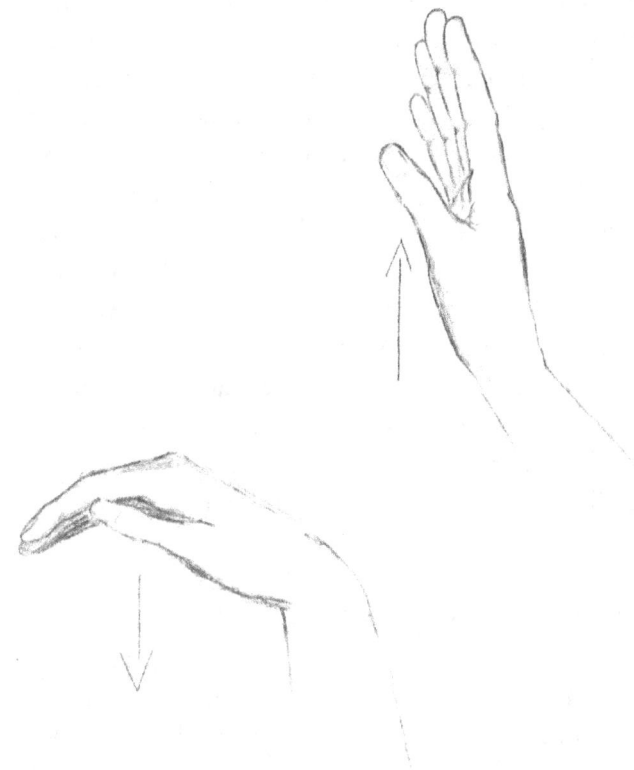

This gesture was not described with words but only demonstrated by Rudolf Steiner. It is very important that the movement upwards and downwards. takes place *between* the tones.

The *rhythmical* element was formed out of the experience that the movement of the quicker tones originates from the front, the lighter side of the gestalt, while the longer tones, which direct us more into our inner being, are held by the back, the darker side of the gestalt. The lightness and darkness were never in relationship to space, neither forwards nor backwards. As with everything musical, even the rhythm lives *within* the human being. (It is different for speech eurythmy, where the human being stands in the outer world.) Some practised the long tones with soul gestures – for instance, longing, expectation, desire, and so on – and the quick tones with small, straightforward movements, originating from the front. We can experience very clearly the difference in the movement of the legs when the gestures are formed with the front or the back of the gestalt. Rudolf Steiner often requested that the long tones be held in their rhythmical quality – if possible, with only one step.

We find this rhythmical experience also in the inner rhythm of the interval forms, which had been given the previous year.[8] They are differentiated so that the tones of the first tetrachord, which are bound to the body, have the character of long tones, while the second tetrachord has a brighter, inwardly quicker rhythm. These forms are to be practised out of the polarity between lightness and darkness, not out of the sculptural element.

Because the musical *beat* has a tendency towards the will, the walking or stepping is affected. The threefold step is thus modified and turned into an inward experience of the difference in character between the left and right side of the human gestalt. This becomes visible in the movement of eurythmy: 'A differentiation may also be shown simply by taking a strong step with the right leg, the left leg being drawn back, before placing it again.'[9]

The weight rests on the right foot during the first part of the bar, while, at the same time, the left is lifted (before the second beat of the bar) and moves towards the right foot (drawing back towards yourself) without placing any weight. Only with the second beat of the bar does the weight shift onto the left foot, thus easing the weight off the right. The beat is

## 5. NEW FOUNDATIONS OF TONE EURYTHMY

not determined by the time signature, be it 2/4 or 3/4, etc., but rather by the addition of the bar line.

All three of these dimensions interpenetrate in every bone, creating a unity, just as in music melos, rhythm and beat express themselves simultaneously in a tone. In this way, it becomes clear that the movements given for beat, rhythm and melos must merge into a unity. But in music, there are countless combinations. How is it, for example, with a tone that is both high and long within a melody?

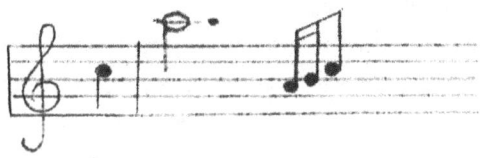

In this case, because the top tone is so high, it is light, but through its lengthy duration, it is dreamy and therefore somewhat dark or passive. It gains, however, an inner strength because it falls on a strong beat of the bar.

In order to give shape to a composition, we must be clear about the character and style of the piece and of the composer. Style and character are expressed in the specific manner in which the three fundamental elements of music – beat, rhythm and melos – are related and connected to each other. The close study of these elements helps us to recognise the basic style of the piece and the characteristics of the composer.

Rudolf Steiner indicated in a conversation with the composer Max Schuurman that beat, rhythm and melos directly mirror the inner constitution of the composer – that is, the relationship of the physical, etheric and astral bodies to each other – while the way in which the bar line is incorporated into a composition reveals the conditions of the composer's incarnation.

With Beethoven, we experience a rebellion, a swelling towards the end of the bar. It is a battle against the bar line. With Mozart, there is a healthy taking hold of the new bar after the bar line. With Chopin, the frequent syncopation and the tendency to constantly start over again point to his suffering and illness. With Brahms, Rudolf Steiner said the bar line is always misplaced because he was not born in the time period belonging to him.*

There is still much to say about this. Just as the colour of the background affects a painting, so does the inner colouring of major and minor always affect the motif in music. In the major mood, will is hidden and one moves with sympathy, whereas in minor, a mood of cognition lives, which draws the movement of the muscles together with a sense of resistance and antipathy.

It is necessary that we consciously grasp the differentiation between tone and speech – whether the 'I' moves outwards or inwards – because the musical element is self-creating, a creation of the human being. We find the musical element in *poetic* speech; for instance, in the 'Wanderer's Nightsong', the lyrical poem by Goethe.[10] Every vowel has its own sound, within which a tone is hidden. In the sequence of vowels given by Rudolf Steiner, the so-called concordance sequence, U-O-A-Ö-E-Ü-I, tones of the musical scale are hidden. When the vowels are spoken through the art of creative speech, it is possible to experience this. In order to achieve certainty and to recognise what is essential in the movement of the interval, it is helpful to discover which 'formative movement' is shared by both the speech sound and the interval – for instance, the Ü and the interval of the sixth.

This divided – connected yet divergent – element of the musical tone and the spoken vowel rests on an unconscious process performed by the soul, namely, to transform what is tone in the human being into vowel.

In a lecture in 1909, Rudolf Steiner said, as a stimulus for a path towards the renewal of the arts:

---

* I heard that he was born a month late. [*Translator*]

## 5. NEW FOUNDATIONS OF TONE EURYTHMY

When you have a melody, you do not only have the single tone, but you also have the overtones with every tone. When you compress the melody into a movement, into harmony, then you do not only compress the single keynotes, but also press all the overtones of all the notes into it. But now the unconscious activity must do something: it must redirect the attention away from the keynotes, in a certain way ignoring them. That is indeed what the soul does, when she perceives the speech sound A (*ah*) or I (*ee*), not as though the other tones were not there, but in a way where the attention is redirected and grasps only the harmony of the overtones. That is the beginning of a speech sound and is how the speech sound arises, when a melody is reduced to a moment and is transformed into a harmony. The keynotes are ignored and only the system of overtones remains. What these overtones produce is the sense of the sounds A (*ah*) or I (*ee*).[11]

The sequence of eight lectures in this tone eurythmy course has itself a similar structure to that of a musical scale. In the first three lectures, we come to know how musical laws find their reflection in the bodily structure of the human organism, and how spirit, soul and body must work together.

In order to grasp the *sense* of melos, Rudolf Steiner guided us a step further to the polar forces of the *Motivschwung* (breath, literally 'motif-swing') and the bar line, both of which live beyond space and time. The musical motif is neither a thought, a representation, nor an aesthetic will that seeks to weave in sounds. The meaning of the motif appears at first as a feeling-sensation for the 'I'. But in order to grasp this meaning, we must behold worlds that we can only divine, that are not only inaudible like the intervals but are worlds beyond space and time. Therefore, Rudolf Steiner again used speech as a means to awaken a feeling for what appears as meaning in the motif.

An anthroposophical lecture cannot be understood if one does not hear the thoughts and feelings that the speaker has during the pauses between sentences and words. The pauses help us to understand what has been spoken. Rudolf Steiner thus led us to an experience of the polar conflict between the spiritually living impulse in the *Motivschwung* (the breath) and the rigidity of the bar line. Both are 'intervals of a different kind' to be found beyond space and time, and they stand in the greatest contrast to each other, like life and death. The *bar line* is lifeless weight, while the *Motivschwung* is the force of will that grasps the incarnating motif. This battle between life and death is fought by the whole of humankind in order to become human. It is the condition for the renewal of life.

In the search for the sense of the melos, which lives between the polar forces of the bar line and the *Motivschwung* or breath, the longing arises to penetrate into the world where the realities of the resounding creative beings are manifested in all their diversity.

In the fifth lecture, Rudolf Steiner provides the foundation needed to grasp these beings who then appear in *choral eurythmy*. Some solo eurythmy movements are modified in choral eurythmy through the fact that the motifs develop their individual form. We must have the courage to leap into a new sphere that is endlessly richer than any virtuosic solo eurythmy performance.

Starting from the element of the *motif,* Rudolf Steiner shows in choral eurythmy how the single motifs appear as beings who are in conversation with each other in space. Time is overcome by the fact that the past, present, and future motifs are simultaneously present. In this connection, the *Motivschwung* or breath is superfluous.

In a solo performance, the *triad* must be transformed into melos in order to be musical; that is, the three tones of the chord must be formed one after the other. But in the choral-eurythmical formation of the harmonies, the individual tones of the chord sound together simultaneously. Here the harmonic principle is at work. The necessity thus arises for the melos, which up until now has been treated only as astral movements in the up-down of the human form, to find its expression in the front-back of the stage space. Also, what was previously given as round and straight forms in space for major and minor, is now valid for the low and high registers of the tones – round forms for the bass and sharp angles for the descant.

The spirit-soul trinity of the chord can be expanded with keynote (tonic), dominant and subdominant to the lofty nine spiritual hierarchical beings who are helpers in guiding the development of the human being.

Difficulties appear in human development through the breaking in of forces that, in music, give rise to dissonances. Dissonances are an alien force that interferes. In eurythmy, the fourth tone erases the appearance of harmony created by the three figures of the triad by moving in front of them – a mysterious process of arising and disappearing again. This erasing can be used in manifold situations, including the erasing of part of a form.

The third indication for choral eurythmy that Rudolf Steiner gave comes out of the rhythmic relationship that lives between the voices. The quicker voices arrange themselves around the slowest tone and create a mobile circling around the voice in the centre. The quicker voice always moves in the periphery. This rhythmical tension in space between the voices must become visible here.

The possibilities given for forms in choral eurythmy appear to be very limited. But we discover that these three basic elements are the archetypal forms for everything that can be created in choral eurythmy. They encompass the whole musical human being in the threefoldness of melos, harmony and rhythm, and they always work together.

But the various principles that had been given the previous year in Stuttgart – for instance, the symphonic presentation with the characteristic forms for the instruments, as well as the interval forms – should not be forgotten.

These indications are archetypes of the musical human being. Archetypes are seeds that can manifest in countless forms and have the greatest possibilities of transformation, just as the archetypal plant, which lives in all species of plants, can always change its form and yet is still the same. All basic forms, in tone as well as in speech eurythmy, should be grasped in this sense.

> Then ... you would be imitating the form of the mighty dance that was performed by the planets and sun in the regions of heaven to make the physical-sensory world possible.[12]

The first five lectures are concluded and completed when Rudolf Steiner helps us through the eurythmy TAO meditation to keep the connection to the archetypal word, to strengthen ourselves in meeting destiny with courage, and to be active in the world with faith in the source of the art of eurythmy. This eurythmy meditation works through the sequence of its intervals and speech sounds, and connects us with the spirit of the earth.

This encounter with the cosmic I-being, the Christ, is the prerequisite for the development of the consciousness soul in the fifth cultural epoch, which, in turn, is needed to progress to the sixth cultural epoch. It is an encounter that depends on the conditions of an individual situation. Therefore, it is also

## 5. NEW FOUNDATIONS OF TONE EURYTHMY

not possible to understand and experience the interval of the sixth without the experience of the TAO. Rudolf Steiner says the following about the TAO:

> You also have to feel the descending progression of notes, and then try to express this in eurythmy, not merely the notes ... and then you will see that in the TAO you have a wonderful means of making your inner bodily nature flexible, inwardly supple, and able to be artistically fashioned for eurythmy ... you will see how by carrying this out you will gain an inner strength which you will be able to carry over into all your eurythmy. This is an esoteric exercise, and when it is carried out it means meditation in eurythmy.[13]

To help us form reliable judgments about which music lends itself to eurythmy, Rudolf Steiner gave us indications about two kinds of rhythms – the *small rhythm* and the *big rhythm*. In the middle ages, they were called *musica humana* and *musica mundana*. Wilhelm Lewerenz explains that the difference between these two rhythms consists in the relationship between the beat and the rhythm of the melody – that is, the difference between the physical and etheric bodies.[14]

In the last three lectures of the Tone Eurythmy Course, Rudolf Steiner turns to a deepening of the foundations. This is, at the same time, an expansion that makes it possible to adapt the movements to the character of the motif.

In order to grasp what is musical in the outer world, we need to overcome our materialistic intellect. For that, we need strong human will. Rudolf Steiner draws our attention to the fact that the will in present-day human beings will become ever weaker through the influence of modern media – cinema, television, radio, etc. – which have a paralysing effect on the will. They generate inner passivity and destroy the possibility of feeling what music is in its full reality.

> The film is the clearest proof that those who like it are unmusical. For the whole basis of films is that they only permit those things to be active in the soul which do not arise out of the inner life of the soul, but which are stimulated from outside.
>
> It must be admitted that a lot of modern music-making tends to lay special stress upon that which is stimulated from outside. Attempts are made to imitate what is external – not by means of the pure melodic element, but rather by employing some subject matter as far remote from the melodic element as possible.[15]

In order to find the musical in the world, Rudolf Steiner gave us an exercise, a kind of meditation. One creates a few sentences with only I (*ee*) and E (as in g*a*te) vowels and other sentences with the vowels U (*oo*), O (*oh*), and A (*ah*). One then speaks them aloud and tries to feel which are musical and which are unmusical. It appears to be a simple exercise, but we are easily led astray. Although everything is clear to the head, and we grasp it intellectually, we do not experience it as reality. This exercise leads us to feel which vowel is appropriate, for example, when a tone is led over into an inward mood or when it is led away from the musical element.

Another exercise is given for grasping the feeling-language of the single motifs in their logical connections. Through this exercise we can gain a unified picture of the soul events in a musical composition. We should take a dream we have had and try to erase from it all pictures, retaining only what arose as soul states of excitement or tension, such as fear, courage, longing, fulfilment, etc. in the sequence in which they appeared in the dream. Thus we reach the reality of the dream, for these same tensions and relaxations could easily have called forth different pictures than those that appeared in the dream. We can also train ourselves to write the dream down in the form of tones. Then we will come to an understanding of the dream.

Once we have enough experience with this process, we can try to decipher the soul language in the motifs of a musical composition. The spiritual content of a composition thereby becomes a self-contained whole, a being that gives expression to its own self. We find the soul colours in the labyrinth of the motifs and are able to work with the composition in eurythmy so that it has a beginning, intensification, climax and a final resolution. The musical composition thus stands before us as a being who brings a message from other worlds. In great compositions – for instance, in those of Bach – the sequence of motifs is often like the progression of a ritual. We can experience through eurythmy how our own 'I' is present both as active participant and as observer.

Nearly all of the practical exercises given by Rudolf Steiner consist of mastering contrasting movements that require and create outer and inner mobility. One example is the exercise of the *sustained note* (pedal point) and the *movement of a rest,* where the constricted and empty qualities of the movement for sustained notes stand in contrast to the activity of the lively, erasing movement of the rests. With a rest, a transition from one world into another takes place. That is why the movement for a rest is related to the erasing movement that arises between the worlds of consonance and dissonance.

This erasing movement for a rest can also be applied in speech eurythmy when the poet changes the direction of thought. After the Speech Eurythmy Course, this was attempted as a group piece based on movements in a circle with the poem 'Nänie' by Schiller. The text itself consisted of

Apollonian forms. Rudolf Steiner asked the speaker to make long enough pauses at the places where the thoughts in the poem were given a new direction.

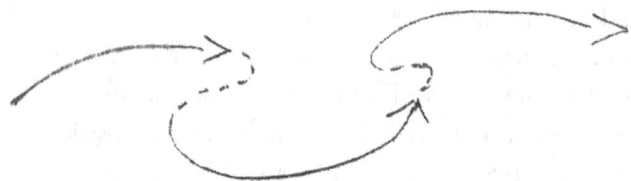

The importance of the in-between erasing movement must be inwardly experienced for it to make an impression on the audience. It is a completion of what has been and a grasping of something entirely new in the next motif of the text.

Two musical motifs without a rest between them require a *Motivschwung*, a breath. But if there is a rest between two motifs, then there must be a slight jolt in the breath, made with the erasing; thus we express the fact that we are going into a spiritual sphere to grasp the next motif. The rest makes the *Motivschwung* more explicit.

In the final lectures of the course, Rudolf Steiner gave the necessary continuation of the first exercises so that we could grasp what is essential in the gestures given for the intervals. The vertical force bestowed on us by the cosmos streams through our arms and hands through the mediation of the collar bone.

> Because movement depends upon making use of these muscles and bones, it is consequently a question of learning to feel how the muscles and bones have to be used in order to do eurythmy in the musical sense.
>
> ... Anyone who is unable to feel at a specific place will never discover the right point of departure.[16]

Without the perception of these forces, the movements of the arms and hands will remain only symbolic signals. But if our consciousness takes hold of the feeling that lives in the muscles and bones, then the interval gestures of the hands will become the visible will-impulse of the spirit.

The interval movements given in lectures two and three remain outwardly unchanged, despite the additional knowledge about the life source from which they originate. The skeleton, which otherwise is the image of death, reveals itself as a hidden source of life.

If we consciously take hold of the collar bone with feeling and connect this feeling with the gesture given for the interval of the prime (the step), then the gesture of the foot acquires its right expression. If this conscious feeling is led on from the collar bone to the humerus, then the closed hand opens in a question, seeking the way to the octave with a far greater expressiveness. If we guide the feeling further, over the elbow into the radius and ulna, then the movement of the third receives its meaning. If we then guide the conscious feeling further through the corresponding bones, then the interval gestures, which would otherwise be only an image, are imbued with their spiritual reality.

If the seventh reaches the octave coming towards it, then 'the octave simply falls into the keynote.'[17] The gesture is the turning of the hand, which clearly shows how the octave comes from the outside and connects itself with the collar bone to the new prime.

If the seventh does *not* reach the octave, the hand remains where it is, lifeless and fixed in space, until the body steps forward along the arm, and, like an in-breath, receives the in-streaming cosmic spiritual forces into the human gestalt. New life, feeling and formative forces fill the human being.[18]

If we descend with the pitch into the depths to the bass tones, then the intervals connect themselves to the coarser bones of the legs, which have the same form as the arms, only somewhat grotesquely distorted. If we look at the skeleton of the arm and leg, we see that the difference between them is like that between a violin and double bass. The muscles and bones of the legs are bound to the gravity of the earth. Rudolf Steiner encouraged us to try to feel the gestures of the legs with the corresponding muscles and bones. Thus, we experience the prime at the starting point of the hip, the second in the thigh bone, the two thirds in the tibia and fibula, the fourth in the heel, the fifth in the arch, the sixth in the toes, and the seventh in the outermost part of the toes. Rudolf Steiner said:

> It is possible to transfer the movements – which we have used to express the notes/tones – to the legs and feet, harder though they are to carry out, and necessarily remaining as an indication. When you transfer the gestures for the notes to the legs and feet, the effect will be less beautiful, but you have here a different means of expression for the legs and feet from dancing, as we have already tried in the most various ways in speech eurythmy and the like.[19]

At the same time, both arms can take on a downward bell-like accompanying movement, which Rudolf Steiner gave as a rhythmical expression, or they can accompany the movements of the legs with the indicated interval movements.

If we try to listen inwardly to the experience of the low tones, a feeling of a great hidden power in these deep archetypal tones arises. We could compare it to the unearthly, terrifying force which announces itself in the depths of the earth before an earthquake or the eruption of a volcano.

Ascending from the bass tones through the seven scales, we experience the whole range of the world of tone. But in

## 5. NEW FOUNDATIONS OF TONE EURYTHMY

every repetition of the seven tones of the scale, there are always different perceptions to be experienced, because we always encounter new spheres that manifest themselves in the tone world with new life sensations.

To bring out the character of the scales in different pitches, it can be helpful to immerse oneself in the lecture in which Rudolf Steiner showed how, during the Lemurian epoch, human beings grasped the whole range of sound through the seven tones, when the distance between notes consisted of ninths: [20] $C_2$, $D_1$, E, F#, G#$^1$, A#$^2$, B#$^3$.

In those times, people had an objective cosmic experience and felt the joy and suffering of the gods. Only in our time did the possibility arise for the seven-tone scale to be an experience of the 'I' within an octave. Today, sense perception goes even further. Not only has the whole audible creation been drawn together into seven times seven scales but some musicians, such as Alois Hába, recognise the quarter tone and use it in their compositions.

The very highest tones of the scale, which our consciousness cannot grasp, can be accompanied by a gentle trembling of the whole gestalt because the whole scale has the character of an out-streaming seventh.

In the spring of 1924, Köhler composed a light piece in which two voices stand in this extreme of high and low registers. Rudolf Steiner couldn't help but laugh when he heard it.

Before Steiner went on to the major and minor cadence, he summarised it briefly:

> The real secret of the difference between major and minor lies in the fact that everything of the nature of major streams out from the will, that is, a streaming-out from the fullness of the human being. Everything that is major is related to *action* (*Tat*). Thus a certain activity must be introduced into all motifs in the

major mood. All phrases in the minor mood are *receptive*. They possess something of *recognition*, of acceptance, of laying hold of something. All phrases in the minor mood are related to feeling. When passing over from a phrase in the major mood to a phrase in the minor mood, we must definitely show that this is a transference of activity from the *outer structure* of muscle and bone to the manipulation of the *inner structure* of muscle and bone in the arm and hand of the eurythmist. It is from feeling and experience of the impulse towards action that all eurythmy has to proceed.[21]

Musical motifs not only flow on and on but can also come to a kind of damming up in the *cadence,* where the flow comes to an end. Just as the sequence of sounds in a simple motif of three notes can become a chord and be expressed through the gesture of the triad, Rudolf Steiner also gives us a eurythmy gesture for the short sequence of chords that form the cadence. It is a concluding gesture in which both arms move from left to right or right to left, according to whether it is major or minor. This movement can even be used when there is only a tendency towards a cadence. It can be done in many ways and is often connected with dissonances or even a fermata or a ritardando. Thus, the erasing before and afterwards (in the dissonance), or the pull to the left with the inclination of the head or shoulders indicating the change in tempo (ritardando), can be carried out in connection with the gesture for the cadence. The tones of the melody can also appear in addition to the sweeping arm gesture for the cadence – for instance, in the angles of the wrist.

We must not forget that, in general, only the essence of the movement was given; the 'how' needs to be developed by us.

We must also make the distinction that the triad is in itself a movement that is carried out in eurythmy forwards or backwards according to major or minor, whereas the cadence, depending on major or minor, finds its expression in the movement from left to right or right to left.

Later on, Rudolf Steiner was shown the movement for the triad in many different zones and even in their inversions with different intervals – for instance, the movement of the four–six chord (second inversion). They were very complicated movements. Unfortunately, these gestures for the chords have been lost, because no one who tried them at the time made notes.

As an introduction to the final lecture, Rudolf Steiner says:

> From yesterday's study, which dealt more with the bodily aspect of the human being, and with the way in which the body is brought into activity in the movements of eurythmy, I should like to pass over today to the aspect of soul, and make clear to you how the life of the soul is brought to expression in every single movement or gesture.[22]

What is meant here by the 'soul element' is the fruit of the work with the previous indications, which arises when one has gained inner experience and outer skill.

The three elements – pitch, duration of tone, and dynamics (forte, piano, etc.) – as well as correct phrasing and the differentiated treatment of the eurythmical forms of the motifs, are the real expressions through which musical feeling itself emerges as the bearer of the 'I', appearing in its soul garment with the many nuances of the sentient soul, intellectual soul, and consciousness soul.

> It is true to say that nothing is musical which is not in some way rooted in human feeling. Similarly, when music streams over into eurythmical movement,

everything which is brought to life in this movement must also be rooted in the feelings.[23]

To avoid any misunderstanding as to what is meant by the 'soul element' of the tone, Rudolf Steiner repeated what he had said the previous year to the teachers of the Waldorf School in Stuttgart.[24] He presented the musical threefold division of the human gestalt: nerve system, rhythmical system and limb system. Within the middle rhythmical organism of the musical human being it becomes: *melos, harmony* and *rhythm*. But this threefold nature is expressed soul-wise in a single tone as: *pitch, duration of tone* and *dynamic*.

What really leads to musical expression is, above all, the *pitch* of the tone. This 'change of position' in the rising and falling, ascending and descending, of the melos must be clearly visible. From this we can see that all movements from below upwards are related to the major experience, and all movements from above downwards are related to the minor condition.

The second element is *duration* of tone or note values, where the tendency of feeling is neither towards thinking, as in melos, nor towards the will. Eurythmists experience the degree of their own inner activity through their capacity to perceive. With the quick tempo they are filled with life and should observe their own movements with interest. With the tones of long duration, they live in a passive, apathetic attitude, with an empty gaze and without interest. In the duration of tone, human beings not only live in themselves, as they do in melos, but, 'in note values a certain enjoyment and participation in the world outside, a contact with the world, exists. A relationship of the human being with the outer world is expressed in note values.'[25]

Although the *dynamic* tends towards the will, it still remains in the realm of feeling. Here the human connection to the outside world is even stronger than in note values. This becomes visible through the tension in the muscles of the hands and arms, which increases as the tone gets stronger until the fingers become pointed in forte and fortissimo, and then finally the arm and foot movements come together with sforzato. When the tone becomes softer, the force in the muscles recedes until the fingers bend inwards with piano and pianissimo.

Rudolf Steiner described to us for the first time the laws for shaping the motifs in three different ways: through repetition, metamorphosis and the introduction of a second motif. The recurring musical motif is an image of certain recurring motifs of destiny that arise in metamorphosed form throughout our life until they arrive at a conclusion, either in victory or defeat.

It is often asked: which orientation should be assumed when Rudolf Steiner spoke of right and left? When he indicated directions in space – in relation, for example, to forms for the repetition of motifs – he always spoke from the perspective of the audience. But when he referred to movements that are carried out in the human gestalt, he appealed to the formative forces as well as to the qualities of soul that are active in a differentiated way in the right and left sides of the human being. This also applies to a fermata, for example, which is accompanied only by a turning of the head towards the left, followed by an immediate turning to the right when the tempo becomes quick again.

If we want to heed all the indications that must be carried out with the whole gestalt, such as the *Motivschwung* (breath), erasing, rest, etc., the only thing that will help us to really differentiate them is an intensive devotion to the character of the mood living in each thing. Then we can form the movements so that they achieve the right expression according to the situation and do not become the same undifferentiated movements, as is so often the case. This necessarily presupposes that we learn to experience right and left, with their different properties and activities, from the perspective of the study of the human being.

In this connection, it is important to remember that Rudolf Steiner always drew forms from the perspective of the audience. Eurythmists have formed the convenient habit of turning the page around – a practice that would be good to overcome. The character of the form can be grasped when we look at it as the audience does. It is also advisable, when creating a form, to draw it as it appears to the audience and not from our own movement on the stage.

In the last lecture of the Tone Eurythmy Course, Rudolf Steiner leaves it to eurythmists to decide whether they want to lead eurythmy further as a new art in the sense in which he founded it. The exercises given are the germinating seeds from which a high art can be resurrected in the distant future.

Thus, we can experience this course as the foundation for a future art of tone eurythmy.

# 6

# Tone Colours

When working with eurythmy, it is helpful to grasp the essence of the different arts. For the muses are sisters who work together, even though each one has her own independent task in world evolution.

Just as a musical composition must have colour and architectural elements, so too, are the elements of the other arts active in eurythmy. But they must be adapted to the nature of eurythmy. A colour, for example, can become deceptive when it appears only as an aesthetic element. To become eurythmical, it must be able to *speak* through its intrinsic colour movement. Goethe's theory of colour helps us to understand this language of colour. He differentiates colours according to their activity and passivity, as well as their intensification. Experiencing colour in this way creates a sure bridge to Rudolf Steiner's insights in his lecture series, *Colour*, which then lead us on to the essential being of colour – for example, to the lustre and shadow colours.

Colour also speaks differently when it comes from the outside, as in lighting, or when it appears out of the inner nature of the human being. We can learn through the study of Rudolf Steiner's lighting indications how, in tone eurythmy, the lighting can be formed according to the element (pitch, rhythm, beat, etc.) that predominates in the composition. In contrast, the lighting in speech eurythmy does not follow the outer mood of the poem in any given moment but, instead, finds expression through a *sequence* of colours that corresponds to the inner tension of the whole poem, as, for example, in Goethe's poem 'Der König von Thule' [The King of Thule].[1]

To understand the colours themselves, it is helpful to study the various indications Rudolf Steiner gave on this theme.

In the finishing school in Dornach, which was founded for girls who had completed their time at school, Rudolf Steiner often gave painting lessons. They were once given the task of painting the zodiac. Signe Neovius-Ljunqvist, who was a student at the time, relates how the zodiac and planets should be painted in the colours given for the *Twelve Moods* in such a way that the colours merge into each other. The circle of planets should be inside the zodiac. And in the flooding colours of the outer circle, the sounds, sound gestures, or the twelve eurythmy gestures for the zodiac should be painted, each in its place. In addition, the animal should be presented in the colour belonging to the opposite sign of the zodiac. Thus, for example, in the red of Aries, the ram itself is painted violet; in the orange of Taurus, the bull is painted light violet; in the yellow of Gemini, the twins are painted light lilac, and so on.

Another task given by Rudolf Steiner to the students at this school was to paint the circle of fifths, using active colours for the sharp keys in the upper part of the circle and passive colours for the flat keys in the lower half. The source of light in the centre of the circle generates both the active colours of the sharp keys ('Light shines through the darkness') and the passive colours in the lower part of the circle ('Light in front of darkness'). Everything was painted in a flowing movement of colour, without boundaries for the single tones, so that with the sharp keys there arises the feeling, 'I brighten the world,' and with the flat keys, 'I take the light into myself.'

## 6. TONE COLOURS

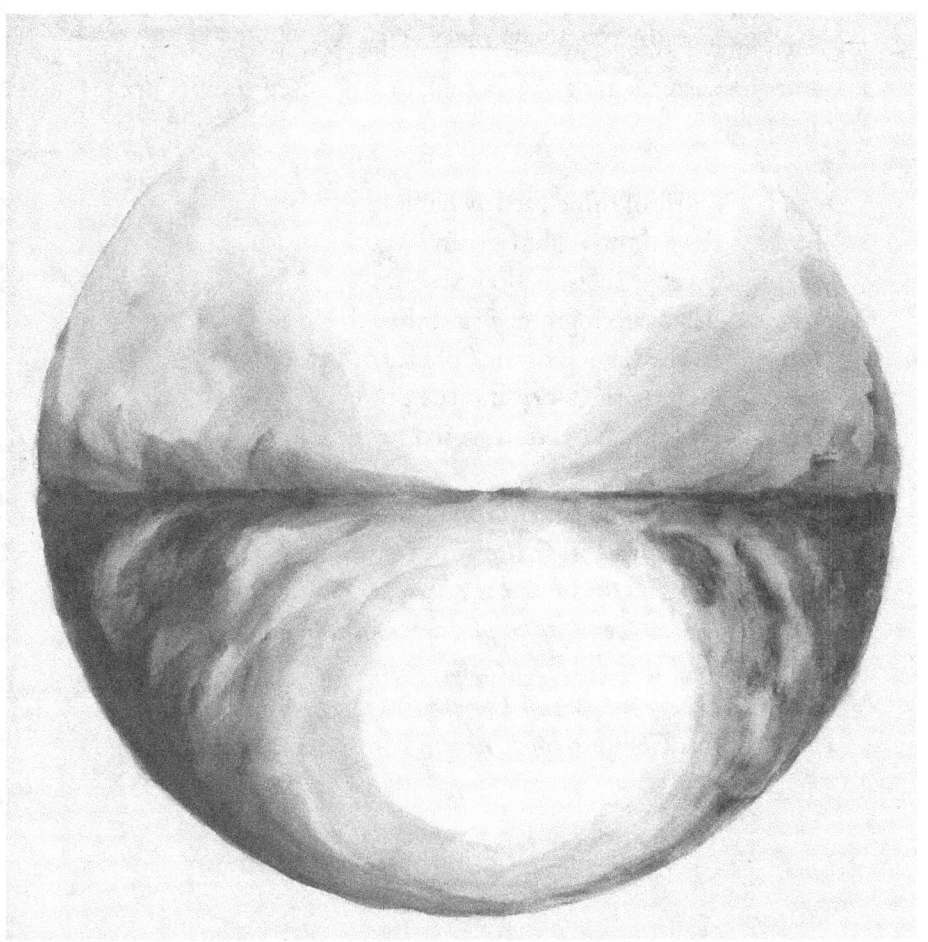

Circle of the Fifths *by Signe Neovius-Ljunqvist who later gifted this painting to the Elena Zuccoli Eurythmy School*
(Colour reproduction on inside front cover)

Rudolf Steiner also gave colours for the scale. In our time, the seven tones of the scale begin with red, which brightens to orange in the second and becomes yellow in the third. The green of the fourth leads to blue in the fifth, which is deepened to indigo in the sixth and appears as violet in the seventh.

Rudolf Steiner gave the following seven-stage verse to someone with the task of experiencing the seven colours in the lines.

| | |
|---|---|
| *red* | Spirit of mine earthly habitation, |
| *orange* | Reveal the Light of thine Age, |
| *yellow* | To the Christ-endowed soul, |
| *green* | That striving I may find thee |
| *blue* | In the Choirs of the Spheres of Peace, |
| *indigo* | Singing the glory and the power |
| *violet* | Of human hearts devoted to the Christ. |

| | |
|---|---|
| *red* | Du, meines Erdenraumes Geist, |
| *orange* | Enthülle deines Alters Licht, |
| *yellow* | Der Christus-begabten Seele, |
| *green* | Das strebend sie empfinden kann, |
| *blue* | Im Chor der Friedenssphären, |
| *indigo* | Dich, tönend von Lob und Macht, |
| *violet* | Des Christus-ergebenen in Menschensinns.[2] |

## 6. TONE COLOURS

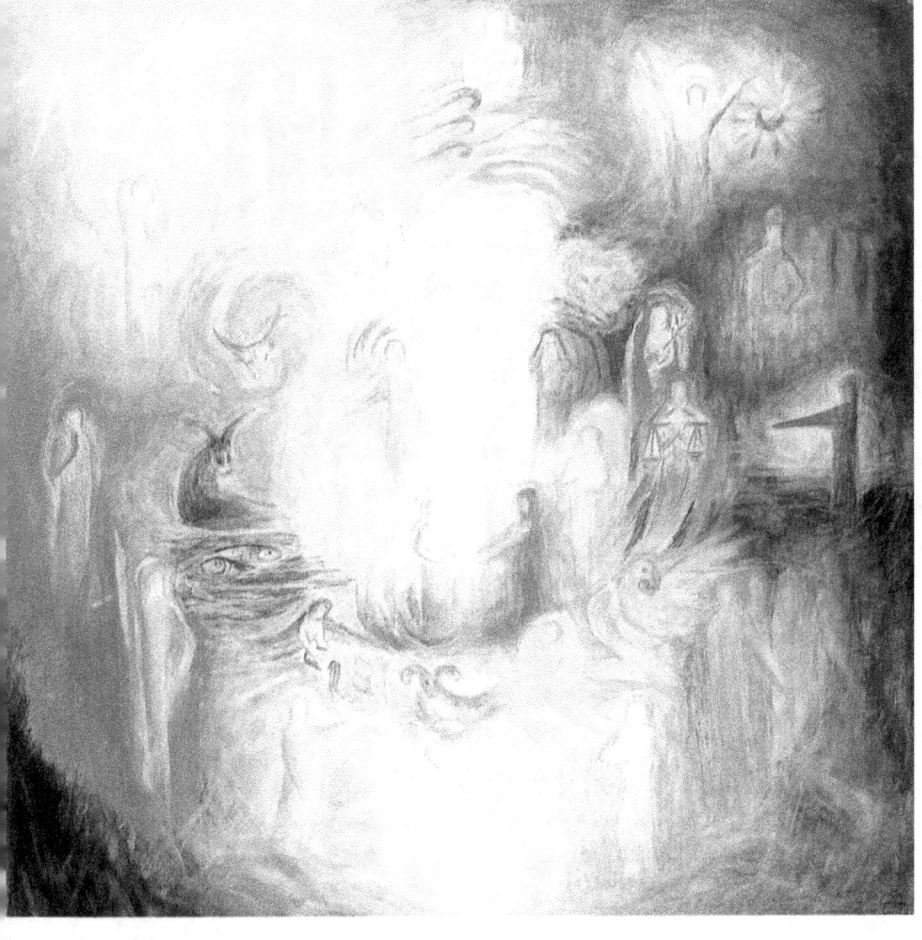

**The Zodiac** *by Elena Zuccoli*
*by permission of Franz Lehnert*
*(Colour reproduction on inside back cover)*

# 7

# The Eurythmy Figures

In 1922, Rudolf Steiner began to create coloured wooden figures, inspired by the attempts of sculptress Edith Marion, to bring the sounds for speech eurythmy into sculptural form. Rudolf Steiner's figures are not sculptural works of art but rather an educational treasure to help eurythmists (and others) understand the etheric in the human being.[1]

The following are excerpts from Rudolf Steiner's lectures that show how thoroughly these indications need to be practised.

> Thus you have a first, fundamental colour that expresses the movement itself, and a second primarily in the veil placed over it, which expresses the feeling. The eurythmy performer must have the inner strength to express the feeling in movement. It is like the difference between ordering someone to do something and making a friendly request. It is in the nuance or level of feeling. Just as an order is different from a request, this second colour – expressed here as blue on a foundation of green – continues into the veil. This represents the feeling nuance in the language of eurythmy.
>
> The third aspect that is brought out is character, or a strong element of volition. This can be introduced into eurythmy only when a performer can experience the

movements as they are made, thus giving them strong expression. The way performers position the head as they do eurythmy makes a great difference in the way they appear. Whether, for example, one keeps the muscles on the left of the head taut and those on the right relaxed – this is expressed here [in another figure] by means of a third colour. You see the muscles on the left of the head are somewhat tense, those on the right relaxed. Observe how the third colour always indicates this here. You see the left side contracted, and down over the mouth. Here [in another figure] the muscles of the forehead are contracted. This, you see, sets the tone of the whole inner character; it radiates from this slight contraction, for this slight contraction radiates throughout the organism. Thus the art of eurythmy is really composed of movement, expressed in the fundamental colour; the feeling nuance, expressed by the second colour; and volition [element of will]. Indeed, volition is the basis of the whole art, but emphasised in a special way.[2]

When you sing, you take into your whole organism – in a physical sense – the elements that move the soul. The movement occurs entirely within the bounds of the skin and remains invisible, flowing fully into the tone one hears.

    The figure you see here (another figure) expresses music in movement. The soul's feeling is released from the human being, becomes spatial movement, and the artistic element is expressed as movement. We see what we otherwise only hear. Thus, these figures are intended only to suggest what a human being becomes while performing eurythmy, completely apart from any natural attributes ... The way eurythmists on a stage manipulate their veils becomes a continuation of the movement. Once eurythmists have learned to do this with skill, the veil will float freely, be withdrawn, caught up, or given a certain form at the right moment. The movement performed by the limbs is behind the feeling that is also expressed by manipulating the veil; the feeling is expressed in the floating veil. If a eurythmist has true feeling for the movement of arms or legs, the quality will naturally pass into the manipulation of the veil, and the feeling that should accompany movement in the veil will be felt.

When this movement (pointing to the figure) is being performed, the eurythmist must be able to sense that the arm is stretched out lightly in this direction, as though hovering in the air with no inner tension. In the other arm, a eurythmist must feel as though summoning all of one's muscular force and packing it tightly into the arm. One arm (the right) is held lightly upward; the left arm is tense, and the muscles almost throb. This is how the movement is given character, and this character makes an impression on the spectators. They can feel what the eurythmist is doing.

Now, when the people look at these figures, they may ask, where is the face and where the back of the head. But this has nothing to do with eurythmy ... You will occasionally find those who are enthusiastic about the pretty face of a eurythmist, but I can assure you that this is not part of eurythmy. The face on this figure, which looks like it is turned to the left, is in fact facing you, and the colour is used to emphasise the fact that the eurythmist should feel 'eurythmic force' diffused lightly over the right side of the head, while the left side of the head is tense, imbued with inner strength. It is as though the head becomes asymmetrical – relaxed, as if 'fluffed out,' on the one side, and taut on the other.

The movements receive their true character in this way. The figures here express what should become visible in eurythmy.[3]

If we look at the thirty-five wooden figures, we find four very differentiated worlds in their laws and characteristics: first, a world of form, which is expressed in the consonants; secondly, the world of the human soul, which works from within, raying out as the vowel element; the third world, which appears as the human soul attitude in thinking, feeling, and will; and as a fourth world, we have the two tone eurythmy figures for the major and minor triads, harmonising with each other in their complementary life of form and colour.

These figures reveal, through their differentiated forms and colours, how life works creatively in the human being. They speak a language that everyone can understand, valid for all human beings.

According to Rudolf Steiner, all colours in the painted figures are to be regarded as shadow colours, as described in the lectures, *Colour*. Someone tried, for instance, to paint the blue in the 'M' figure as though it were a lustre colour. The effect was that the veil appeared to be a separate entity that did not belong to the speech sound.

What appears as *movement* in the figures is the etheric body of the human being. Rudolf Steiner shows at the beginning of the first lecture of the Speech Eurythmy Course (*Eurythmy as Visible Speech*) how the collective movements of the sounds of the alphabet produce the etheric gestalt of the human being. As such, this etheric body is invisible to the senses, and the task of eurythmy is to make it visible, through movements, as an image of the Word in the human being.

With the consonants, the colour and form of the veil are united with the movements of the arms. The arms sculpt in the veil the forms of feeling living in the speech sounds. Here, *feeling* becomes form.

The *character* of the sound appears in the etheric gestalt, that is, in the movement itself. Here eurythmists are asked to understand the language of colour within the will. They must differentiate the colour according to whether it appears as movement, feeling, or character. Green, for example, is at rest in the *movement* of the impact sound 'M', but in the *character* of the sound 'R', it acts decisively as a halting process, as a restraining force, so that a circling arises in connection with the red of the *movement* and the yellow of the *feeling*.

It is noteworthy that none of the sounds have green veils but only some of the soul gestures, which points to a hardening of the soul, for example, in the soul gesture for 'question' or to a growing inflexibility in human feeling as in 'damned clever'.

Because the vowels are a soul-spiritual expression originating from the inner human being, the *movement* is already an element of soul, and the interplay of the colours is different than in the world of form connected with the consonants.

We notice, first of all, when looking at the figures for the vowels, how the arms form a unity with the whole gestalt. And we also see how the veil follows the *movement* freely and, for the most part, is not bound by the physical arms. But this does not exempt the eurythmist from having to give form to the inner, invisible feeling so that the audience can perceive it, even though it does not appear physically.

When we place the figures for the vowels in the order in which Rudolf Steiner spoke about them in lecture six of *Eurythmy as Visible Speech,* the colours of the *movement* of the vowels are in the sequence of the rainbow: violet, blue, green, yellow, red; A (*ah*) – U (*oo*) – E (*ay*) - I (*ee*) – O (*oh*).*

If we examine further how it is with the *feeling* colours, appearing in the vowels only as a form of sensing, it is astonishing to discover that we find only lustre colours, which in the painting of the figure are obviously applied as shadow colours:

| the radiance (lustre) of the spirit | yellow | E, O, U, |
| the radiance (lustre) of the soul | blue | A |
| the radiance (lustre) of life | red | I |

The colour of the *character* of the vowels appears only in the duality of warm and cool colours, red and blue, and in their combination as violet:

| red | A, E |
| violet | U |
| blue | O, I |

Or, we can say that in the will region of the vowels, the past appears in A (*ah*) and E (*ay*) as red, while in O (*oh*) and I (*ee*), the blue leads us into the future. In between is U (*oo*) with violet.

In every vowel figure we can also recognise in its three colours how the self, the 'I', determines the relationship between thinking, feeling, and will. And we can discover in

---

* *Purple* (reddish lilac) has something expanding towards which the blue sky comes (greenish, bluish veil).
*Blue* has a forming quality that strives towards one's own star (yellow veil).
In *green* light and dark meet, my 'I' holds itself upright opposite the spirit of the world (light yellow veil).
*Yellow* (yellow orange) radiates; I have found power to live in aliveness (red veil).
*Red* (reddish) my 'I' expands itself to lustre of life, towards loving embrace of the world; I have become active in the radiant glory of the spirit (greenish yellow veil).

## 7. THE EURYTHMY FIGURES

the relationship of the colours a new law showing how the sentient soul, the intellectual soul, and the consciousness soul arise.

From this point of view, all the vowels reveal the following law: in every figure, there are two colours in opposition to each other, but the third colour holds the balance between them. For example, in the vowel A (*ah*) we have the contrast of red and blue in the *character* and *feeling*, while the red-violet in the *movement* has the connecting power. We can also say that with the A (*ah*), the *movement* of the etheric thinking controls *feeling* (blue) and *willing* (red). A (*ah*) is the representative of the intellectual soul. Before us stands the cosmic Astrid as she appears in Rudolf Steiner's Mystery Drama, always in the A-position.

Thus Philia can also be experienced through the fact that the polar forces of the I (*ee*) – the warm yellow of the *movement*, which rays out from the centre, and the blue of the *character*, which leads from the periphery inwards – find their equilibrium and their master in the red of *feeling*, where both forces hold the balance. The task of every vowel can be grasped in this way.

The relationship of the three colours is pronounced only in the vowels. It can perhaps also be found in individual consonants but not as an underlying law.

The difference between the consonants and the vowels becomes clear when we compare two that have corresponding colours, for example, B and I (*ee*). Both have radiant yellow dresses. In B, the arms are formed by the blue feeling, but in the I (*ee*) both arms follow the yellow-orange of the movement.

When we consciously shape this different treatment of the veil in the form-world of the consonants and the soul-world of the vowels, we can see in the eurythmic movement how language is permeated by the planetary and zodiacal forces.

In all the figures for the soul gestures (in which the four temperaments can also be found) the harmonising of the three colours is focused on a *condition,* and the colours support each other in the same direction. The basic character of these gestures originates from sympathy and antipathy, as developed at the end of lecture six of the Speech Eurythmy Course (*Eurythmy as Visible Speech*). The soul gestures are attributes of the human being and live in human thinking, feeling, and will, which can be discerned through the colour of the *movement.* When we place the wooden figures of the soul gestures in the sequence in which Rudolf Steiner introduced them in lectures five and six of the course, we discover whether they belong to thought, feeling, or will according to the colour of the dress.

The first group of figures all have light (predominantly yellow) colours for the movement; they belong to human thinking. The second group of figures have either greenish or reddish colours for the movement; they reign in the world of human feeling. And the third group of soul gestures are anchored in the human will and have blueish colours for the movement. It is only the figure for Communication that is placed between the groups of feeling and willing, although it has a yellow colour for the movement. In this figure for Communication, the red colour of the will acts as fervour, eagerness, and enthusiasm; the violet colour of the feeling wants to expand from behind forwards in 'restrained will'; and the thoughts in the 'moved posture' are radiant yellow.

In the same lecture, he challenges eurythmists, when creating forms for a poem, to seek out the soul gestures that correspond to the content of the text and then to use the Dionysian forms for thinking, feeling, and willing according to these soul gestures. The soul gestures bring into the movement the mood expressed in the voice – for example, a loving or commanding mood.

## 7. THE EURYTHMY FIGURES

To show how a vowel can become a soul gesture, in lecture five, Rudolf Steiner demonstrates the sound I (*ee*), which in a choleric temperament becomes 'self-assertion or almost megalomania'. We can follow the process in the transformation of the colours. The red veil remains in both, but instead of being behind, as in the vowel I (*ee*), the red appears in the front in 'almost megalomania'. The blue of the will in I (*ee*) becomes black, and the yellow of the movement in I (*ee*) becomes green.

With the appearance of the first eurythmy figures in 1922, the colours, tensions, and forms were practised diligently. Tatiana Kisseleff achieved mastery with them and insisted that no sound gesture be done without the colours. It was difficult to acquire the skill of grasping, throwing, and releasing the veil, of giving it the corresponding shape while having the tension of the will in the head and feet. The sounds V, B, S, and T were nearly always formed with the veil, which we grasped with the hands. This work with the figures deepened the work in speech eurythmy.

Mastering the colours of the sounds happens much more quickly than one would imagine. In time, one discovers how the movement of the individual sound can be differentiated.

Many questions have been raised in connection with the eurythmy figures for the major and minor triads, which are the last two figures Rudolf Steiner created in the summer of 1924 and which were shown to us for the first time during the Speech Eurythmy Course. Sometimes they are considered as the cadences, but then he would not have written the triads on the back but instead the cadence sequence as it was played in the Tone Eurythmy Course when he spoke about the cadence.[4]

From these two figures we can see what the colour tells us in the element of beat: in major, red is the carrying fire, and in minor, green, the complementary colour, is the arresting, weighing down quality.

When choosing the dress and veil for a piece of music, it can be helpful to know, through observing the figures for major and minor, that the melos is expressed in the dress and the rhythm in the veil. The colour of the beat remains hidden but is visibly present as the retarding or carrying force.

We must never forget that colour is movement. In the Speech Eurythmy Course, we experienced an example of how rigidly we view the eurythmy figures as finished positions. When, in lecture six, Rudolf Steiner spoke about the wooden figure for High Ceremony (or Ceremonial Festivity), which was standing in front of him on the desk, its arm was exactly as on the original sketch, directed to the right. Now, he spoke continuously about the movement of High Ceremony, how it goes from right to left. We became increasingly restless until Rudolf Steiner noticed our unrest and said, 'Yes, it is indeed the case that here the movement forms itself from right to left; there is no mistake here.' It goes from the position of Knowledge on the right over to the left into High Ceremony. Since then, this movement has also been done on the left side, in mirror picture to the sketch. Rudolf Steiner did not see anything wrong with having drawn it on the right.

We find a similar problem with the minor figure. If we follow the movement of the veil colour for the two triads as described in the first lecture of the Tone Eurythmy Course, then the movement of the veil colour of the minor figure can convey that the gesture for the minor third comes back towards the gestalt.

# 8

# Speech Eurythmy

This chapter only makes a few comments about the Speech Eurythmy Course, *Eurythmy as Visible Speech,* given in the summer of 1924.

There was great activity on the Dornach hill. The last remnants of the wall of the first Goetheanum had been torn down and ground into gravel that was used to improve the pathways around the building. Walking on them made one ponder: how much more deeply would Rudolf Steiner's words have affected us if the lecture course could have been held in the great hall of the first Goetheanum? Its colours and forms would have been unforgettable examples to the eurythmists – for everything in the Goetheanum was formed out of the etheric world.

All of the eurythmists who were able to travel to Dornach had come for the course. In the first row of the auditorium in the carpentry shop sat the still quite young eurythmists, who nevertheless belonged to the 'old guard', ready to step up onto the stage to demonstrate what had been spoken about. The many interruptions created difficulties for the stenographer, and, therefore, a number of indications and important remarks by Rudolf Steiner were not included in the shorthand report.

The mood in the hall was festive. One felt that Rudolf Steiner's words were imperishable realities. To begin with, he tried to clarify for us what the etheric body is, and then he placed about twenty questions in front of us. These questions are the steps on the path of knowledge that leads to the source from which the creative forces always arise anew. They form the path for the eurythmist to develop self-knowledge and to come to know the Word from which everything originates, inspiring us with its call to action.

In his second lecture the following day – after speaking about the essential nature of the eurythmical consonants and vowels, and correcting and renewing some of the movements – Rudolf Steiner strengthened the feeling in the audience that the sounds of speech apply to all languages.

Originally, there was a single unitary language spread over the whole earth. Through the fact that human beings went through a process of individualisation, and because the Word thus became more and more bound up with the individual, many different languages arose – the Tower of Babel is an image of this. Because the 'I' entered into human beings, individualised thinking, feeling, and willing could also arise within them.

Rudolf Steiner then led us into the world of human soul attitudes that are conditions of the soul, as are, for instance, the four temperaments. Here he showed us the wooden figures of the soul gestures, which are prototypes for etheric movement.

Further on in the course, he led us into the world of 'becoming and dying away'. In this etheric realm, the elemental forces hold sway, but these forces should not be confused in eurythmy with their physical appearance in fire, air, water, and earth. In the elemental life of the world of birth and decay, the four types of consonants are differentiated. With the gestures for the *impact* or *plosive sounds,* the forming of the sound becomes visible through the movement that precedes it, whereas with the *fricatives* or *breath sounds,* the existing form of the sound is dissolved or dispersed. Thus, one has the impression that the impact sound is in a state of becoming, while the breath sound is dying away. The forming of the impact sound ends with a 'stiffening of the muscles'. The opposite happens with the fricatives, where the existing form of the consonant is dissolved as the upper body follows the movement of the arms. This phenomenon is clearly audible in the echoing of the air when speaking a breath sound, whereas the preceding movement of the impact sounds is inaudible and happens etherically.

R and L, which also belong to this becoming and dying away, take place in the inner realm of the human being. Rudolf Steiner indicated that, for the sound R, the body should move 'beautifully with a swing up and down', and that L should be formed 'rhythmically with a swing forwards and backwards, right into the physical'. With L, the forwards and backwards motion of the body starts in the ankles, whereas, in the R, the knees determine the rising and falling of the gestalt.

The impact sounds have an inherent element of egoism in their forming quality, while the fricative sounds have an inherent element of surrender to the surroundings into which they die away.

If we observe these laws in the eurythmical world of the consonants, we undergo a process of purification in regard to the influence of Ahriman and Lucifer. These two can be active in the sounds if a eurythmist, out of a certain sense of ease and comfort, makes all of the movements uniform. The movements will always be interesting when eurythmical differentiation is practised and when every consonant can find its rightful place in the world order.

In lectures two to eight, Rudolf Steiner characterises all of the sounds almost three times, but each time differently, enriching them through new perspectives, going from the single sound to the word. Throughout these lectures he continuously swings back and forth between consonants and vowels. This can be an important indication for eurythmy teachers.

In lecture nine, Rudolf Steiner leads us further into imaginative, poetic, pictorial language, where metaphor and synecdoche* are found – metaphor in the eurythmic spatial movement of right and left, and the synecdoche in the movement forwards and backwards. Rudolf Steiner employed metaphor and synecdoche in all his eurythmy forms. Knowing this helps us find the correct division of the text on these forms.

During the tenth lecture, Rudolf Steiner announced a surprise:

> Today we will take our start from the nature of man, endeavouring to discover the forms that may arise out of the nature of man. Then, moving on somewhat further, we shall ask ourselves, 'Which sound is to be regarded as related to this or that corresponding form?'[1]

This was the climax of the course. Every gesture shows the image of a divine origin and becomes for us a 'divine teacher' through its gesture, which we have to translate into movement. These gestures form the new twelvefoldness of the 'human circle' that became possible through the event of Golgotha, replacing the Egyptian zodiac of the third cultural epoch. Already in 1915, through the text of the *Twelve Moods* given by Rudolf Steiner, and through the indication of the twelve colours for the veils, there were signs that a new circle is coming into being.†

---

* A figure of speech where a term for the part is used to represent the whole.

† For a long time, Rudolf Steiner had wanted to create new signs for a zodiac appropriate to our time. For the first edition of the *Soul Calendar* of 1912, twelve pictures for the months were created, under Rudolf Steiner's direction, by the painter Imma von Eckhardtstein. In 1924, when a new edition of the *Soul Calendar* was to be published, Rudolf Steiner was asked whether the twelve zodiac pictures from 1912 should be included, and he answered that he himself wished to draw new pictures. Unfortunately, he did not find the time for this.

## 8. SPEECH EURYTHMY

The all-encompassing remark at the beginning of lecture twelve is important:

> The first thing I would like to discuss is how (as we have seen) certain moral impulses that we placed before our souls in the numbers twelve and seven are expressed in human gestures, in gestures that are held and in gestures that move. That is, it is just as possible with eurythmy to think that one can come to conclusions out of the soul's experience – that is what we are dealing with here – or having come to a conclusion one can also enter the experience, and that then flows into the sounds.[2*]

After Rudolf Steiner had connected the earthly language of sound to the spirit of the human being, he could show us, through various practical examples, how the art of eurythmy thus contains a further possibility for development.

He invited four eurythmists onto the stage and asked them to demonstrate the well-known 'I and you' exercise while facing the front and taking on the following four gestures of the zodiac before and after the text: Taurus, Leo, Eagle (Scorpio), and Aquarius.

---

\* Ralph Kux related: 'Especially fresh in my memory is the exceptional liveliness he [Rudolf Steiner] displayed during the Speech Eurythmy Course. For instance, when he showed us the forms for the movement of the zodiac, he got onto the stage with the lightest step and showed every eurythmist the characteristic movement that they should do for the respective zodiac sign. Glowing enthusiasm lay in his eyes and gestures as he moved with youthful elan amongst the artists. One had the impression of a great teacher who wished to ignite drive and power for the deed' (Kux, *Erinnerungen an Rudolf Steiner*).

Ralph Kux was an exceptionally spiritual human being, extremely taciturn and quiet, and a very talented musician and eurythmist. He composed a great deal for eurythmy and directed large eurythmy performances at the Goetheanum, including *Job*. He died immediately after a rehearsal in December 1965.

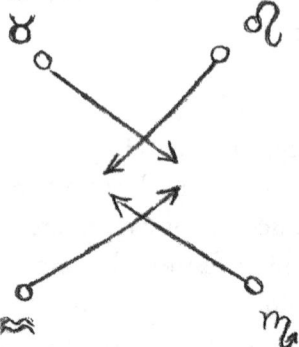

With the last words, 'are we', the human being is shown in their moral qualities. That is, one is only a whole human being when head, heart, and will have united in harmony.

In addition, the *Peace and Energy Dance,* which was given very early on, was developed further in its expression through a change in tempo. It is important to note that Rudolf Steiner clothed the exercise in words to show how texts can be treated rhythmically.

| Strive for peace | *Strebe nach Frieden* |
| Live in peace | *Lebe in Frieden* |
| Love (the) peace | *Liebe den Frieden* |

This text (the last three lines of the *Peace Dance*) has of necessity a discrepancy in the German language between the thought and the will, because the rhythm of the words is dactylic while the meaning of the text has an anapaestic mood. In eurythmy, the dactyls must be transformed into anapaest stepping so that the rhythm is suited to the thought.

One often finds that the rhythm of the language does not correspond to the content. That presupposes an intensive study of the different rhythms so that one can recognise their characteristic expression.

## 8. SPEECH EURYTHMY

We also achieve a harmony between thinking, feeling and will through the metamorphosis of form, as, for example, in the three forms given for the Hallelujah. With the pentagram, which was known, the movement is carried out in the calm mood of thinking. With the crown form, this mood unites itself with feeling, and finally, through the addition of curves in the third form, the process is intensified into willing. The Word imbues the whole human being in that it grasps the heart by thinking and leads to deed in the will.

The rhythmic element commands a broad range of activity and has many possibilities of expression. The simple stepping of rhythms with poetic speech already brings the audience into a soul-etheric world. But rhythm can also be applied in forming sounds for characteristic elements, as indicated, for example, by Rudolf Steiner for the beings that appear in the 'Classical Walpurgis Night' in Goethe's *Faust*, Part II. There, for instance, the two sphinxes should only do eurythmy with the arms on the unaccented vowels of the text. That gave the impression of endless wisdom-filled calm and granite-like weight.

The Apollonian forms, given by Rudolf Steiner in 1915, grasp the individual words and are to be felt like an occult script. It does not appear to be a coincidence that in the Speech Eurythmy Course in 1924, the zodiac precedes the Apollonian forms.

The basic exercise that goes from sound to sound in the zodiac unites the different forces of the zodiac in a single word, and the words that arise in this way are taken up by the Apollonian forms as if into a vessel.

With a further step into the Apollonian world, we encounter the grammatical laws of nouns, adjectives and verbs, which are the requirements for building a sentence, and we also encounter three different circles. These are generally known only as the basic forms that Rudolf Steiner gave for the *Dance of the Planets*. The circles reveal the heavenly origin of grammar as sun, moon and planets.

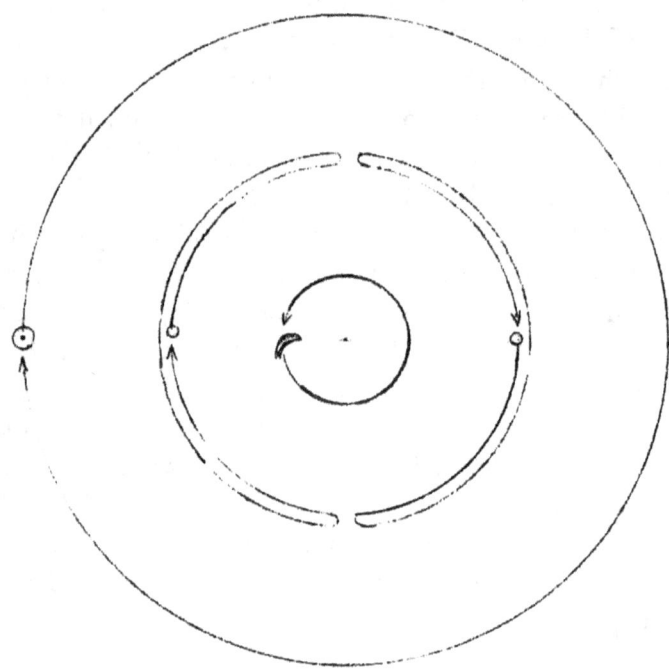

The *nouns* belong to the outer circle, the sun circle. They are sun beings because they are only tangible when light is present – physical light for concrete objects, soul light to feel the inner soul life, and spiritual light to grasp thoughts.

What we perceive as light is a purely spiritual element that is perceptible to the senses, in contrast to the force of gravity, which is an invisible sensory phenomenon.

In this course, Rudolf Steiner amended the names of the nouns to distinguish their different qualities because the previous names, 'abstract' and 'concrete', were easily misleading. He divided the nouns into five groups.

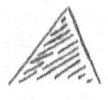 *1. Sense-perceptible objects*

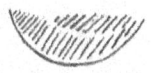 *2. Spiritually perceptible, such as inner picture, idea, phantasy*

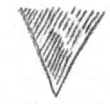 *3. The conditions that adhere to outer objects, such as the red of the rose*

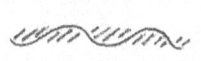 *4. Qualities held entirely in the soul, such as love and faith*

 *5. Spiritual beings, such as Michael, God, Lucifer*

Rudolf Steiner drew the five forms of the nouns and filled them in to show clearly that they are not lines of movements, as they appear in all other eurythmy forms, but rather that they are like vessels for the form (*Gestalt*) of the word.

With the *verbs,* which are moved on the innermost circle, the straight line is the directive for the eurythmist. For here the line is not, as in the Dionysian forms, an image for the paths of thinking, but rather the expression of the creative quality that we can experience when we step sideways, forwards or backwards. The verb has a moon quality in the sense that the moon forces are the driving force in all that grows or is secreted. Thus, the moon forces are active in speech in all the movements of the verbs and also in interjections.

In the middle circle between sun and moon, the other five planets appear. This circle carries all the adjectives, adverbs, pronouns, etc. In their restrained movement they give the nouns and verbs their specific character and thus connect being and action.

Forming speech on these three circles demands of the eurythmist a wide-awake consciousness of the whole. What sun, moon, and planets say must be experienced side by side. Only then does a unity arise, as can happen in an ideal social form. It is the same experience we have when looking at the starry heavens.

The question arises: is it possible that the *Dance of the Planets* by Rudolf Steiner is an example of how one can work with Apollonian forms in a different way? This poem is composed in such a way that the first line can be regarded as a noun, the second and third lines as more adjectival, and the fourth line as having the quality of a verb. Thus, this poem is a grand example of how Apollonian principles can be applied, not pedantically but imaginatively in broad strokes.

It is essential to experience the difference between how the *Twelve Moods* and the *Dance of the Planets* should be performed. In the verses of the *Twelve Moods*, every planet has its own circle (seven circles within the circle of the zodiac), and the transitions between the stanzas are carried out simultaneously by all seven planets (the moon stands, holding the centre). The text is done in standing (with the exception of the sun). In contrast, in the *Dance of the Planets*, the planets are on one circle – here, too, the circles are divided into twelve parts – and every planet forms the gestures *with* the text as it moves along the circle from one zodiac sign to the next. It is the mood that lives *between* the twelvefoldness, like in an interval. It gives expression to what is happening between the constellations.

This holds good for the different possibilities that have been given for the *Dance of the Planets*. If one varies the *Dance of the Planets* – for instance, having twelve eurythmists for the sun circle – the division of the four lines remains the same, but the line for the sun is always divided between two eurythmists. For example, in the first line of the first verse: Aries functions as the consonants, Taurus as the vowels. In the sun line of the second verse: Taurus now functions as the consonants, Gemini as the vowels, etc. In this version, the sun line is done in standing.*

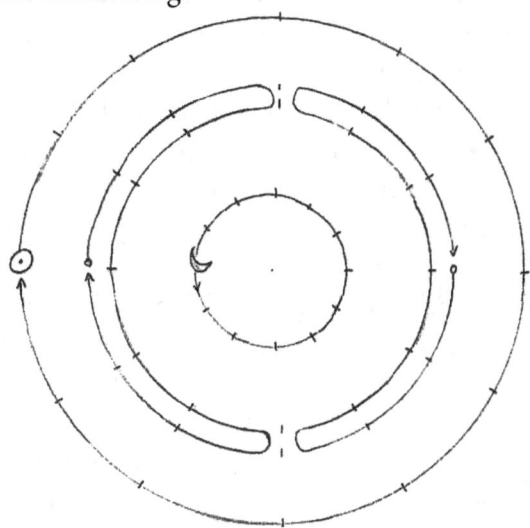

In both verses, the eurythmy zones remain the same – that is, Aries and Libra in feeling, and Cancer in thinking. With Scorpio, the arm movements enter the will sphere below the shoulders and are completely submerged in Capricorn; they then rise a little higher in Aquarius, while still remaining below the shoulder. Only in the last line of the *Twelve Moods* – 'Let loss become its own gain' – do the arm movements rise all the way up.

It was Rudolf Steiner's wish that whenever the *Twelve Moods* is performed the satire *The Song of Initiation* also be included. It is important to remember that the satire belongs to present-day humanity. The words of this text are spoken satirically by Ahriman about Lucifer.

* It is noteworthy that in the *Dance of the Planets,* the sun has a red veil, the moon, as always, a purple veil, one of the planets a green veil and the other a blue veil – the latter two pointing to Venus (green) and Saturn (blue) as representatives for the inner and outer planets.

The Cosmic Introduction also consists of three circles and a transition to the next place, meaning the forms live in the movement of time. Rudolf Steiner advised that this be taken up as a preparatory mood for the microcosmic 'Larynx'. This latter form has three semi-circular platforms on which the sounds of the alphabet are distributed and shows how the cosmic forces of the sounds of speech are related to thinking, feeling, and will within the microcosm.

On the *topmost step*, the vowels, all diphthongs, and the straight lines of the Apollonian forms (verbs, sense-perceptible nouns, and conditions) are expressed. The whole human being arises – that is, the soul element of the vowels unites with the will (verbs) and the gestalt (nouns). On the *second step*, everything adjectival is done in standing, in addition to some of the consonants. On the *lowest step*, the rest of the consonants are carried out, as well as all round Apollonian forms for the abstract (spiritually visible) nouns, spiritual beings, and qualities of soul.

Rudolf Steiner also gave the indication to present the thinking element on the three steps according to the relationships of thought: on the *topmost step*, the main thought; on the *second step*, the continuation belonging to it; and on the *lowest step*, the concluding thought. As an example of such a distinction of thought, Albert Steffen's poem was given: 'Warum hat nicht Kraft, uns zu vereinigen'.[3] The attempt was often made to work with this poem as a group form, but it was never satisfying. It only worked on the three steps described here.

The platforms can also be used for dramatic works. Rudolf Steiner encouraged this, for instance, in the Mystery Drama scene of the conversation in Devachan between Maria and the Soul Forces with their choruses.[4] Scenes from Greek dramas, such as those by Aeschylus and Sophocles, can also be done on the three steps. But here the platforms are shaped like parabolas and not like the microcosmic semicircles.

## 8. SPEECH EURYTHMY

The scope of Apollonian forms is vast, and they can be handled in various ways. For example, when used not in a solo but in a group form, it is possible to create an impersonal and completely objective quality by making a 'form in standing' with many people, who then move to the next form *between* the words. It is the same principle that was given for the Pater Noster, the Lord's Prayer in Latin. The challenge here is that the movement really appears between the words. It is necessary to have the impulse for the next movement already in the last syllable, in order to stand still before the sound of the next word. There arises the alternation between 'movement without arm gestures' and 'standing with arm gestures'. The clearer this alternation between legs and arms is, the more interesting it becomes. A soul gesture can also be formed if the speaker gives enough time between the words.*

To enhance the experience of the polarity between Apollonian and Dionysian principles, it is good to practise in eurythmy what Rudolf Steiner describes in his lectures on architecture. In the Greek Mysteries, the earth motif as bud and the sun motif as blossom were alternately carried by the people in a procession.[5] The bearers of the bud motif responded to all of the Dionysian sentences, while those carrying blossoms responded to everything expressed in an Apollonian way. The bearers of the bud experienced how the forces from the depths streamed through them, through their arms and hands, into the bud, with the tendency to bring the bud to blossoming, while the Apollonian bearers of the blossom carried the light of the cosmos into the gestalt.

Every work of art is permeated by Apollonian and Dionysian qualities. An example is the poem by Albert Steffen 'Die Sonne Fliegt.'[6]

---

* For the Pater Noster (Lord's Prayer) as group form (Apollonian), we used the same forms that Tatiana Kisseleff received from Rudolf Steiner as a solo form. They can be found in Kisseleff's book, *Eurythmy and Rudolf Steiner*.

Apart from the Apollonian, Dionysian and standard forms, Rudolf Steiner gives us various forms for the spiritual beings Philia, Astrid, Luna, Ahriman and Lucifer. The very first forms that were given are like signs that grasp the fundamental character of the beings and reveal their individual nature.

The three soul forces, Philia, Astrid and Luna, which convey cosmic feeling, cosmic thinking, and cosmic will within the human being, have received specific gestures in addition to the forms. Philia, with the vowel sound I (*ee*) – as the feeling – connects the upward-streaming forces with the rising movement of the eyes, head and arms. She has no form, and the eurythmy should be done in standing because feeling is a process in the inner realm. Astrid with the vowel sound A (*ah*) connects sense perception with cosmic thinking. She has the form of a lemniscate, the iambic rhythm, and the lowered position of the head with a downward gaze, while the gestures are carried out in the horizontal plane of the circumference. With Luna, who manifests the self or 'I' of the human being in the world and establishes the consciousness soul, the 'I' *strides into the world* with the cretic (amphimacer) spondaic rhythm, with the gaze turned outwards and straight ahead, while the arms form the gestures below in the region of the will.

Ahriman and Lucifer received their characteristic solo forms at the very beginning of eurythmy. When we connect the first three forms for Lucifer – lemniscate, moon and circle – it is remarkable that the activity works its way from inside out, for Lucifer likes to be seen. With the forms for Ahriman, it is the opposite. From the first spatial form, only a line remains, gradually vanishing into nothing. Ahriman's movement is fleeting and shadow-like, whereas Lucifer is full of light and egoistically enjoys his own movements.

# 8. SPEECH EURYTHMY

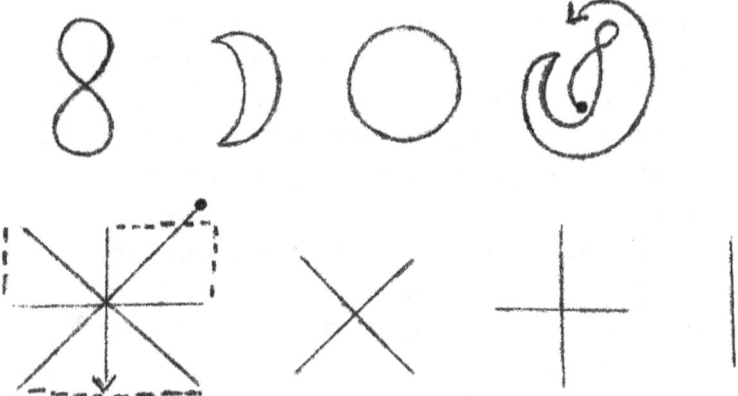

*Above: forms for Lucifer. Below: forms for Ahriman*

The last admonition that Rudolf Steiner gave eurythmists is contained in the Letter to the Members, where he summarises the essentials of the Speech Eurythmy Course.

> Eurythmists need devotion to the smallest of gestures so that their presentation really becomes the natural expression of the soul. They can only form the large gestures when the smallest first become conscious and then become the natural expression of the soul being.
> ... In eurythmy, one can learn the technique of the art; but one can also be deeply permeated by the fact that the technique strips away everything external and must be grasped by the soul if the truly artistic element is to come alive. In all fields of art, people often say how the soul must work *behind* the technique; in truth, the soul must be active *in* the technique.
> ... Eurythmists cannot separate themselves from their artistic creation and place it objectively before the onlooker like a painter or sculptor, but remain personally within their presentation. In eurythmists one sees whether art lives in them as a divine reality or not ...

This course sought to help the participants come to an understanding of this fact. It sought to show how, by watching the gesture, the feeling is ignited in the soul and how this feeling then leads to the experience of the visible word. We can reveal through eurythmy gestures much that can only be expressed imperfectly in the audible word. The audible word in recitation and declamation, brought into connection with the visible word, gives a total expression that can bring about the most intensive artistic whole.[7]

We had a lot to digest after the course. Above all, the new spiritual positions of the zodiac posed many problems that needed to be overcome through practice.

Rudolf Steiner had somewhat exaggerated the gesture for Aries to show what was meant: the stretched index finger pressed against the chin. It was a symbolic gesture for looking back on one's own deed. All six of us entered the stage with this gesture for the Whitsun verse 'Creature ranks with Creature in the Widths of Space' (*Wesen reiht sich an Wesen im Raumesweiten*).[8] It looked very odd. Marie Steiner requested that we soften the gesture. We tried various things until there arose the gesture of the straightened vertical hand below the chin. But this gesture shows something quite different. It emphasises the upright force of Aries (which it also possesses) but not the aspect of looking back on one's own deed. Over the years, the Aries gesture has corrected itself, but one still often sees this somewhat Egyptian gesture. With the gestures for Virgo and Pisces, the bending of the left arm is often too similar. In Virgo, the arm is held firmly against the hip bone at the side, whereas with Pisces, the bent arm is further forward and points towards the right foot, which stands in connection with the right arm stretching upward.

# 9

# Costumes

During Rudolf Steiner's lifetime, art, above all, prevailed in Dornach. Everything was concentrated on the Goetheanum building and on eurythmy. There were performances every Sunday, and often every other day during conferences, with new pieces added to the programme. The art of music was also nurtured and belonged to the realm of eurythmy. Until 1925, only a small eurythmy stage group existed in Dornach, under the direction of Marie Steiner. There was as yet no group of actors. Nearly all the costumes, lighting, and eurythmy forms were drawn and designed by Rudolf Steiner. The task of shaping the programmes lay in Marie Steiner's hands, and the choice of texts depended on the ability and artistic possibilities of the participating eurythmists. Choosing pieces that are suited to the task is the first step towards the success of a programme. Sometimes a eurythmist wanted to try out a piece of music or a poem of her choice, but already in the first rehearsal it was not accepted because either the piece or the artistic capacity was not suited to the aim of the programme.

The question is often asked, 'Why are trousers not suitable for a eurythmy costume?' This question reveals the lack of clarity about the fact that eurythmy movements are etheric. The etheric body has no skeleton; bones belong to the mineralised aspect of the human being. Trousers emphasise the contours of the physical bone structure. When Rudolf Steiner indicated using trousers in the costume for 'The Critic', a humoresque poem by Goethe, it was because he wished to indicate the withered etheric body.

For the 'Clown's Song' in Shakespeare's *As You Like It*, trousers are also indicated, but they are so puffed up with scraps of veil and richly adorned with colourful strips of silk that they no longer have the character of trousers. They are much more a fantastical creation that allows for strong movements of the legs, which would not be possible with a dress.

The costume indications we received from Rudolf Steiner were often different from what one would expect, and we learned that the costume should only support the movement of eurythmy. It was astonishing how he was able to call forth the essential aspect of the thing by very simple means and to awaken the imagination of the audience. When the lighting was added, the whole became a work of art.

The basic form of the eurythmy dress is given as the TAO form. For those who want to know more specifically about the first eurythmy dress, indications for it can be found in the drawings by Tatiana Kisseleff in *Eurythmy and Rudolf Steiner*.

The dress for women went down to the ankle and that for men went to the calves. In the very beginning, dresses with short sleeves were worn, but the veil reached the wrist. The dresses made partly of cotton were used because they do not cling to the body and do not reflect the light like silk. Cotton is more appropriate for some roles – for instance, animals in fables, but also many other figures. In the *Fugue in B-flat minor* by Bach, the indication is for five cotton dresses without veils. Everything that emphasises the outer form of the body in any way had to be avoided because the etheric body consists only of movement and has no fixed shapes.

## 9. COSTUMES

Many years later, with the costumes for animals, indications of the animal's head were added; but, unfortunately, this is the love for naturalism, which is exactly what should be overcome. It directs the attention of the audience away from the expression of the gestures. The imitation of the outwardly visible animal should also in no way enter into the eurythmic movement. Instead, the expression of the soul qualities of the animals should appear. An example of this is the wolf. As the only animal costume given by Rudolf Steiner, it received a turban that was thicker in the front, giving the impression that this creature hides something untrue in its thoughts.

All head coverings are difficult when they draw attention to themselves, instead of supporting the eurythmic movement. Later attempts, such as gold crowns, for instance, in 'Ariel's Scene' in *Faust*, or flowers for the elves in *A Midsummer Night's Dream*, are a disturbance. Such things hamper the gestalt and destroy the expression of the arm movements. Here, too, we must forego much and only indicate the essential nature of the being in question.

Dresses divided into two colours can be good for figures who are of a divided nature, such as good citizens in whom thinking and will do not unite or where the feeling is too weak.

Some dresses were also painted; for instance, for Chinese poems. There flowers were indicated with light yellow strokes on a light blue cotton, giving the impression of brocade.

At the time, there was no choice between thick and thin veils as there is today. Thin veils only came onto the market after the Second World War. For both speech and tone eurythmy, the corners of the veils were rounded so that the veil could follow the arm movement unhindered. When no specific indication was given, they varied only in length – long for speech eurythmy and short for tone eurythmy.

The short veil for tone eurythmy strongly emphasised the rhythmical system of the human gestalt, and the arms also appear to be longer. By contrast, in speech eurythmy, the veil emphasises the vertical direction – the will and the thought element.

All the veils had the same thickness as those used today for the *Soul Calendar* veil. These take on the colours of the lighting much more intensely. The veil also covered the cord at the waist, making the whole torso nearly invisible.*

How the veil should be pinned was left quite free and depended on the artistic needs. Once, during a costume rehearsal, a eurythmist arrived holding a loose veil in her lifted arms. She had come late and had not found time to pin the veil to the dress. Rudolf Steiner felt that it was also possible to make sounds in the air in this way but remarked that the veil must be attached to the dress in one place. This made doing the gesture for E (as in g*a*te) difficult, and he advised her to throw both ends of the veil into the air at the same time from one hand to the other to achieve the crossing of the veil in the air. This was practised a lot and used in 'The Eagle' by Robert Hamerling.

In Rudolf Steiner's humoresque 'Der Erfrorene' (the frozen one), the loose white veil should be allowed to fall to the ground at the end.

The opinion is prevalent that the diagonally pinned veil was Rudolf Steiner's indication for male eurythmy costumes. But this way of pinning the veil originated from a particular situation in which a woman was performing the male role of a knight in a poem. There was the desire to differentiate this from the costume of the elves, who had the veil pinned in the usual manner covering two arms. This was the origin of the diagonal pinning that stemmed from the concept of a toga. Rudolf Steiner's indication was that the *left* side is covered by

---

* At that time coloured cotton cords were used for belts (*Translator*).

the veil, and it should not be done the other way around. The indication that was given only for men's costumes was that the veil should be short like the tone eurythmy veil but have ample material so that some of the veil extended above the arms. This was hardly ever used because it was difficult to control the extended part of the veil in such a way that it responded to the movements and did not just hang limply down. The men refused to wear it.

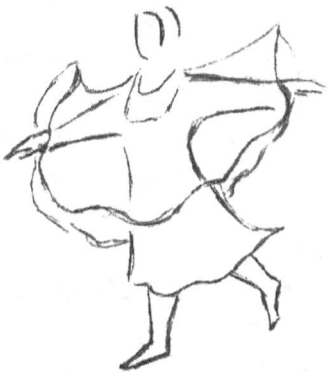

*The men's veil extending above the arms*

Alice Fels, the director of the first Eurythmy School, later said that in 1922, Rudolf Steiner told her to make sure the veils were worn right from the beginning, from the very first eurythmy lesson. She had to argue that the school was poor, for it was the time of inflation. Rudolf Steiner responded by saying she should then hang cloths over the arms. But it appears that this was also a problem. The experience of many years of teaching has shown that Rudolf Steiner's advice was sound. An objective gesture could have arisen with far greater force had this advice been followed. The difference in how the form of the word and the sound of the speech work together – the weight of the earth and the forming power of air – would have become more self-evident. If the foundation is not laid from the beginning, it is far more difficult to achieve this later.

At first, Rudolf Steiner himself applied the makeup to the eurythmists, but everyone feared this because it definitely did nothing for their beauty. His way of applying makeup allowed the head to appear in harmony with the rest of the gestalt.

He gave us principles for the makeup for eurythmy that do not apply to actors. The eurythmist is an image of the etheric, and as much as possible everything of a bony nature must disappear and gain life. Therefore, to everything of a bony nature in the face, red was applied, also to the ears if they were visible. Otherwise, they are very distracting. The peculiar thing is that it does not appear red to the audience, but rather the forehead, nose, and everything bony appears to be penetrated with life, and one appears younger. Sometimes the hands were also slightly reddened, but that became too risky for the veil and dress.

In the summer of 1924, Rudolf Steiner gave the advice at the end of a conversation with Emica Senft-Mohr and the musician Jan Stuten to make masks for eurythmy. Unfortunately, neither attempted it immediately, nor did they ask for more exact guidance. Emica Senft designed the first mask in 1926, after Rudolf Steiner's death when it was too late to receive help. There were many technical problems until she took the eurythmy figures as her starting point and imitated the shape of the head with stiffened, coloured gauze. Because the material was transparent like tulle, she did not need to make holes for the eyes, nose, and mouth, and it was very pleasing, this expressionless face, which was much more expressive than the formed physiognomy. The big problems that remained were the transition from the mask to the dress, as well as the proportion of the head to the whole body, because the head always appeared too big. In other respects, this seemed to be a possible way forward.

## 10

# Eurythmy Work with Marie Steiner

It was 1926. After the turbulence of the first summer conference without Rudolf Steiner, there were lingering reflections and strong criticism as the result of all the preparations and performance. In spite of everything, the work of the eurythmists continued without pause.

Now actors came to Dornach in order to put into practice the Speech and Drama Course, which Rudolf Steiner had given two years previously at their request.

At that time, Marie Steiner was still connected with our daily work with eurythmy, and in this working together she tried to help us along with new impulses. Through her, many large eurythmy compositions for the stage had already arisen – among others, the *Fairy Tale of the Green Snake and the Beautiful Lily* by Goethe. This was the first attempt at a fairy tale, and the question arose, 'Can one do eurythmy to prose?' But this text of Goethe's fairy tale is so poetical that the prosaic is overcome.

She had also tried to compile texts out of Rudolf Steiner's lectures on the Hibernian mysteries to present images of an initiation on the stage in eurythmy. This period of collaboration was a very beautiful time.

Marie Steiner had an exceptionally good command of the Italian language, of which she was very fond. She had attended the readings of the poet Giosuè Carducci in Italy over a long period of time. One day, she asked me whether I would be willing to do something in eurythmy in the Italian language, which she would gladly recite for me. As I had worked on Dante for a time and tended more towards the dramatic element, I chose the death of Count Ugolino in Canto XXXIII of the *Inferno,* the Count being a character who is especially famous for his language. I went to work with great joy. During practices without a speaker, I helped myself by means of the echo that was exceptionally good in the Brodbeck House.* I spoke and used the echo as speaker. Soon I was ready and approached Marie Steiner, who immediately settled on an evening when she was happy to try it out.

The large hall of the Carpentry Shop was empty and dark. The only light came from the rehearsal light on the stage and the reading lamp that stood on the little table next to the big armchair. The chair stood on the platform in the middle of the hall. Marie Steiner always directed us from there. We were both, each in our own way, full of anticipation and expectation. She briefly glanced at the text and then began. I had heard many recitals of Dante, but now it was quite new. The dark space filled itself with enormous speech-images. Her voice grew ever stronger, and I felt as though the whole Carpentry Shop was trembling. It grew more and more, and I had to gather all my forces to keep up with her formative power. Suddenly, she shut the book and said, 'Zuccoli, we may not go further here.' She explained that this was because eurythmy may not come into contact with the subhuman element. Only the beginning up to Canto V of the *Inferno* could be done in eurythmy. I am very grateful for this experience.

---

* The practice room was in the cellar of the Brodbeck House (Rudolf Steiner Halde) in Dornach.

## 10. EURYTHMY WORK WITH MARIE STEINER

In the early years, when the large stage of the second Goetheanum was finished, every Sunday a eurythmy performance was given in which Marie Steiner attempted to realise various indications by Rudolf Steiner. Thus, she tried to further develop *silent* eurythmy. She chose the *Soul Calendar* verses with *Vortakt,* text and *Nachtakt.*

Through a spoken text, it is natural for there to be a common experience. Through musical accompaniment, a unity in the group is also achieved. But with silent eurythmy, this unity is very difficult to attain, especially when the participants have different sounds, as is the case in the *Vor-* and *Nachtakts* of the *Soul Calendar* verses. Thus, the task given by Marie Steiner was a difficult test for us. The audience also had a problem understanding and were left unsatisfied.

Only after the Second World War was this theme taken up again. Through the performance of Rudolf Steiner's seven Planetary Seals, in which the evolution of the earth becomes visible, interest for silent eurythmy was aroused in the audience.* One could see that it was easier for the audience to take in the eurythmy movement 'in and of itself' without recitation.

Today, visible speech in silent eurythmy has yet to be achieved. But we can sense the power it could have if it were.

---

* Elena Zuccoli created eurythmy forms for Rudolf Steiner's Planetary Seals.

We want to bring the spirit, which is in us as a seed, to blossom and fruit so that we can find the gods again.
　*Rudolf Steiner,* Die Impulsierung, p. 57.

# Notes

## 1. The First Impulse in 1915
1 See Steiner, *A Psychology of Body, Soul, and Spirit,* lecture 3, Oct 26, 1909.
2 Steiner, *Links Between the Living and the Dead,* lecture 2, pp 43–45.
3 Steiner, *The Inner Nature of Music.*
4 Steiner, *Eurythmy: Its Birth and Development,* p. 160.
5 Steiner, *The Inner Nature of Music.*
6 Steiner, *Eurythmy as Visible Singing.*
7 Steiner, *Eurythmy as Visible Singing,* lecture 1, p. 42.
8 See Steiner, *Eurythmy: Its Birth and Development,* pp. 101–8, and Kisseleff, *Eurythmy and Rudolf Steiner.*

## 2. Reawakened Interest in Tone Eurythmy
1 Steiner, *Eurythmy: Its Birth and Development,* p. 122.

## 3. The Birth of the First Eurythmy School
1 Steiner, *The Inner Nature of Music,* lectures 5 and 6, March 7–8, 1923.
2 Steiner, *The Inner Nature of Music,* pp. 64, 67f.
3 Steiner, *The Inner Nature of Music,* p. 71.
4 Steiner, *The Inner Nature of Music,* pp.72f.
5 Steiner, *The Inner Nature of Music,* p. 68.

## 5. New Foundations of Tone Eurythmy
1 Steiner, *Eurythmy as Visible Singing,* lecture 1, p. 38 (emphasis added by Zuccoli).
2 Steiner, *Eurythmy as Visible Singing,* lecture 1, p. 40.
3 Steiner, *Eurythmy as Visible Singing,* notebook entry for lecture 2, p. 141.
4 Steiner, *Eurythmy as Visible Singing,* lecture 2, p. 50.
5 Steiner, *Art as Seen in the Light of Mystery Wisdom,* lecture 2, p. 41.
6 Steiner, *Eurythmy as Visible Singing,* lecture 2, p. 52.

7 Steiner, *Eurythmy as Visible Singing,* lecture 3, p. 61.
8 See Steiner, *The Inner Nature of Music.*
9 Steiner, *Eurythmy as Visible Singing,* lecture 3, p. 66.
10 O'er all the hilltops / Is quiet now, / In all the treetops / Hearest thou / Hardly a breath; / The birds are asleep in the trees: / Wait, soon like these / Thou too shalt rest. (Tr. Henry Wadsworth Longfellow)
11 Steiner, *A Psychology of Body, Soul, and Spirit,* lecture 3, Oct 26, 1909.
12 Steiner, *Art and the Theory of Art,* lecture of Oct 28, 1909, p. 50.
13 Steiner, *Eurythmy as Visible Singing,* lecture 5, p. 89.
14 The distinguished musician and composer Wilhelm Lewerenz, who later was the first to succeed Marie Steiner as leader of the Section for the Performing Arts, gave me an excerpt from his lecture of April 21, 1943, 'Die Musik und der Auferstehungsgedanke' (Music and the resurrection thought):

Since ancient times, we have had the threefoldness of melody, harmony, and rhythm. When tones appear one after the other, it results in the element of melody. If they sound simultaneously, the element of harmony appears. These are the two fundamental pillars of music. But this is something that is not musically alive; rhythm is missing. Now we must separate rhythm and beat.

... Beat is the simple periodicity. The essence of beat is that the same strokes ... recur at regular intervals.

Rhythm, in contrast, is a living movement. Rhythm is an expression of life. Now, in classical music, beat and rhythm are often in such a close connection that one could consider them equivalent. Therefore, the musician must differentiate between *small rhythm* and *large rhythm.* The small rhythm originates from the movement of the human body and is therefore an expression of the *musica humana.* If one intensifies this rhythm, it can go through various stages, but the last intensification is ecstasy.

It was an exceptional learning experience when Rudolf Steiner heard about attempts I had made in this direction and made clear to me why the small rhythm (where beat and rhythm have a very close connection) should be avoided, especially when music is meant for eurythmy. He added: 'In time, this rhythm should not be allowed to come into the hands of eurythmy.'

Rudolf Steiner showed this again in two pieces of music that were then being performed in eurythmy. The one is a beautiful movement from a sonata by Mozart (Andante from the Piano Sonata in F major KV 283) is an example for the small rhythm; the other a piece by Bach (*Prelude in F minor, Well-Tempered Clavier, Book 1,* No. 12) is an example for the large rhythm.

The movement by Mozart he designated as uneurythmical in this context, whereas the piece by Bach as very eurythmical.

Mozart has, of course, many compositions that are very eurythmical, just as Bach has many compositions that are in this sense not

NOTES                                                                 121

eurythmical. The indication relates in a specific connection only to
music. Rudolf Steiner gave characteristic movements for a part of this
Mozart piece.

All art connected to Rudolf Steiner's work has quite different starting
points and a different goal than what is wished for by the general
audience of today.

15 Steiner, *Eurythmy as Visible Singing,* lecture 6, p. 92.
16 Steiner, *Eurythmy as Visible Singing,* lecture 7, pp. 101f.
17 Steiner, *Eurythmy as Visible Singing,* lecture 2, p. 52.
18 See the description of the descending seventh in Steiner, *Eurythmy as Visible Singing,* lecture 3, p. 59.
19 Steiner, *Eurythmy as Visible Singing,* lecture 7, p. 105.
20 Steiner, *The Inner Nature of Music,* lecture 7.
21 Steiner, *Eurythmy as Visible Singing,* lecture 7, p. 108 (emphasis added by Zuccoli).
22 Steiner, *Eurythmy as Visible Singing,* lecture 8, p. 113.
23 Steiner, *Eurythmy as Visible Singing,* lecture 8, p. 113.
24 Steiner, *The Inner Nature of Music,* lectures of March 7 and 8, 1923.
25 Steiner, *Eurythmy as Visible Singing,* lecture 8, p. 116.

## 6. Tone Colours

1 See Steiner, *Beleuchtungs- und Kostümangaben.*
2 Steiner, *Verses and Meditations,* pp. 192f. See also Steiner, *The Destinies of Individuals and of Nations,* pp. 8f.

## 7. The Eurythmy Figures

1 Steiner, *Entwürfe zu den Eurythmiefiguren.*
2 Steiner, *The Spiritual Ground of Education,* lecture 8, pp. 117f.
3 Steiner, *A Modern Art of Education,* lecture 12, pp. 194–96.
4 Steiner, *Eurythmy as Visible Singing,* lecture 8.

## 8. Speech Eurythmy

1 Steiner, *Eurythmy as Visible Speech,* lecture 10, p. 111.
2 Steiner, *Eurythmy as Visible Speech,* lecture 12, p. 130.
3 ('Why' does not have the power to unite us) in Steffen, *Wegzehrung.*
4 See *The Portal of Initiation,* scene 7, in Steiner, *Four Mystery Dramas.*
5 See Steiner, *Architecture as a Synthesis of the Arts,* lecture of June 7, 1914, p. 59.
6 (The sun flies) in Steffen, *Wegzehrung.*
7 *Nachrichtenblatt,* July 20, 1924, in Steiner, *Eurythmie; Die Offenbarung der Sprechenden Seele.*
8 Steiner, *Verses and Meditations,* pp. 82f.

# Bibliography

Kisseleff, Tatiana, *Eurythmy and Rudolf Steiner: Origins and Development 1912–39,* tr. Dorothea Mier, Floris Books 2021.

Kux, Ralph and Willi, *Erinnerungen an Rudolf Steiner* [Recollections of Rudolf Steiner] Mellinger Verlag, Stuttgart 1976.

Steffen, Albert, *Wegzehrung* [food for the journey] Verlag für Schöne Wissenschaften, Dornach 1983.

Steiner, Rudolf. Volume Nos refer to the Collected Works (CW), or to the German Gesamtausgabe (GA).

—, *Architecture as a Synthesis of the Arts* (CW 286) tr. Johanna Collis, Rudolf Steiner Press, UK 1999.

—, *Art and the Theory of Art* (CW 271) tr. Dorit Winter and Clifford Venho, SteinerBooks, USA 2021.

—, *Art as Seen in the Light of Mystery Wisdom* (CW 275) tr. Pauline Wherle and Johanna Collis, Rudolf Steiner Press, UK 1984.

—, *Beleuchtungs- und Kostümangaben für die Laut-Eurythmie. Deutsche Texte I: Ägyptisch bis Goethe* [Lighting and costume indications for speech eurythmy. German texts I: from Egyptian to Goethe] Rudolf Steiner Verlag, Switzerland 1980.

—, *Colour* (CW 291) tr. John Salter and Pauline Wehrle (Forest Row, UK: Rudolf Steiner Press, UK 1997.

—, *The Destinies of Individuals and of Nations* (CW 157) tr. Anna Meuss, Rudolf Steiner Press, UK 1986.

—, *Die Entstehung und Entwicklung der Eurythmie* [The origin and development of eurythmy] (GA 277a) Rudolf Steiner Verlag, Switzerland 1998.

—, *Entwürfe zu den Eurythmiefiguren* [Sketches of the Eurythmy Figures] (GA K 26) Rudolf Steiner Verlag, Switzerland 1984).

—, *Eurythmie. Die Offenbarung der Sprechenden Seele* [Eurythmy: the revelation of the speaking soul] (GA 277) Rudolf Steiner Verlag, Switzerland 1999.

—, *Eurythmy as Visible Singing* (CW 278) tr. Alan Stott, Rudolf Steiner Press, UK 2019.

—, *Eurythmy as Visible Speech* (CW 279) tr. A. Stott, C. Schmandt, and M. Stott, Anastasi, UK 2015.

—, *Eurythmy: Its Birth and Development* (CW 277a) tr. Alan Stott, Anastasi, UK 2002.
—, *Eurythmy Therapy* (CW 315) tr. Alan Stott, Rudolf Steiner Press, UK 2009.
—, *Four Mystery Dramas* (CW 14) tr. Ruth and Hans Pusch, SteinerBooks, USA 2014.
—, *Die Impulsierung des weltgeschichtlichen Geschehens durch geistige Mächte* [How spiritual powers give impulses to historical events] (GA 222) Rudolf Steiner Verlag, Switzerland 1989.
—, *The Inner Nature of Music and the Experience of Tone* (CW 283) tr. Maria St Goar, Anthroposophic Press, USA 1983.
—, *Links Between the Living and the Dead* (part of CW 140) tr. D.S. Osmond and C. Davy, Rudolf Steiner Press, UK 1973.
—, *A Modern Art of Education* (CW 307) tr. Jesse Darrell, Anthroposophic Press, USA 2004.
—, *A Psychology of Body, Soul, and Spirit* (CW 115) tr. Marjorie Spock, Anthroposophic Press, USA 1999.
—, *Speech and Drama* (CW 282) tr. Mary Adams, Anthroposophic Press, USA 1960.
—, *The Spiritual Ground of Education* (CW 305) tr. Christopher Bamford, SteinerBooks, USA 2004.
—, *Twelve Moods* tr. Ruth Pusch, Mercury Press, USA 1984.
—, *Verses and Meditations* (CW 40) tr. George and Mary Adams Rudolf Steiner Press, UK 2004.

## Works by Elena Zuccoli

*Eine Autobiographie,* Verlag am Goetheanum, Switzerland 1999 (not translated).
*Aus der Toneurythmie-Arbeit an der ersten Eurythmie-Schule in Stuttgart, 1922–1924,* Verlag Walter Keller, Switzerland 1980 (published in English as *From the Tone Eurythmy Work at the First Eurythmy School in Stuttgart 1922–24,* but long out of print).
Available works by Elena Zuccoli can be found at:
www.eurythmeum.ch/shop-downloads.html

# Index

A *(ah,* vowel) 47f, 59
adjectives 99
adverbs 99
Ahriman 104f
Apollonian element, forms 16, 97, 104
Astrid (in Mystery Drama) 87, 104

Bach, *Fugue in B-flat minor* 108
balance 14
bar line 58, 60
Baumann-Dollfuss, Elisabeth (1895–1947) 45
beat 54, 56
Beethoven, Ludwig von (1770–1827) 48, 57
blue 86
Brahms, Johannes (1833–97) 58
breath (fricative) sounds 92f
Bruckner, *Eighth Symphony* 32, 39

cadence 70f
Carducci, Giosuè (1835–1907) 114
Ceremonial Festivity (eurythmy figure) 90
Chopin, *Prelude in C minor* 35
Chopin, Frédéric (1810–49) 58
choral eurythmy 60f
Christmas Conference 1923/24 43f
colours
—, lustre 84
— of eurythmy figures 81f, 84
— of tones 75–78
—, shadow 84, 86

Communication (eurythmy figure) 88
consonants, character of 87
Corelli, Arcangelo (1653–1713) 48
Cosmic Introduction 102
costumes 107–11
— for animals 109
cotton (for dresses) 108

*Dance of the Planets* 16, 98, 100f
Dante, *Inferno* 114
Deventer-Wolfram, Erna van (1894–1976) 20, 45
Dionysian element, forms 16, 104
Dollfuss, Elisabeth Baumann- *see* Baumann-Dollfuss
dresses
—, painted 109
—, two coloured 109
Duncan, Isadora (1877–1927) 13
dynamics 72f

E *(ay,* vowel) 48
Eckhardtstein, Imma von (1871–1930) 94
etheric body 107f
Eurythmy School, Stuttgart 31–33, 42

Fels, Alice (1884–1973) 31, 111
fifths, circle of 76f
figures, eurythmy 81–90
—, colours 81f, 84
film 64
fricative (breath) sounds 92f

gesture for rising or falling tone 55
Goethe, *Fairy Tale* 113
—, 'The Critic' 108
green 86

Hába, Alois (1893–1973) 69
Hamerling, Robert (1830–89) 110
—, 'The Eagle' 110
head coverings 109
Hibernian mysteries (lectures) 113
High Ceremony (eurythmy figure) 90
Hollenbach, Hendrika (1881–1950) 25–27, 29
humoresque 110

I (*ee*, vowel) 48, 59, 89
iambic rhythm or steps 28
I-A-O exercise 48
impact (plosive) sounds 92f
intervals (musical) 37, 49
—, prime 50, 67f
—, second 50, 68
—, third 47, 50, 68
—, fourth 38, 50, 68
—, fifth 37, 51, 68
—, sixth 37, 51, 58, 68
—, seventh 37, 50, 67f
—, octave 51f, 67
—, ninths 69
Italian language 113f

Jenny-Schuster, Maria (1907–2009) 44

Kisseleff, Tatiana (1880–1970) 25, 89, 103, 108
Köhler, Hedwig (1890–1940) 31–33, 35, 40, 43, 69
Kux, Ralph (1903–65) 95

L (sound) 93
Laban, Rudolf (1879–1958) 13
languages, different 92, 113f
left 73
Lewerenz, Wilhelm (1898–1956) 63, 120
lighting 75, 107f

Ljunqvist, Signe Neovius- *see* Neovius-Ljunqvist
Lucifer 104f
Luna (in Mystery Drama) 104

Maier-Smits, Lory (1883–1971) 14
major mode 19, 27, 47–49, 69, 72
major tones, long 28
—, quick 28
makeup 112
Marion, Edith (1872–1924) 81
masks 112
melos 22, 54
metaphor 94
minor mode 19, 27, 48f, 70, 72
minor tones, long 28
—, quick 29
Mohr, Emica Senft- *see* Senft-Mohr
*Motivschwung* (breath) 59f, 66
movement (of vowels) 85f
Mozart, Wolfgang Amadeus (1756–91) 57
music lectures 33
*musica humana* (small rhythm) 63
*musica mundana* (big rhythm) 63

*Nachtakt* 115
Neovius-Ljunqvist, Signe (1905–75) 76f
note, sustained (pedal point) 65
nouns 98f

O (*oh*, vowel) 48

*Peace and Energy Dance* 96
Philia (in Mystery Drama) 87, 104
pitch (musical) 72
Planetary Seals 115
plosive (impact) sounds 92f
poem, forms for 88
purple 86

R (sound) 93
red 86
rest, movement of 65
rhythm 54
—, big (*musica mundana*) 63
—, small (*musica humana*) 63

# INDEX

right 73
ritardando 70

Sakharoff, Alexander (1886–1963) 13
satire 101
scale(s)
— of whole tones 18
—, major 19
—, minor 20f
—, seven 68f
Schiller, Friedrich (1759–1805),
 'Nänie' 65
Schuster, Maria Jenny- *see* Jenny-
 Schuster
Schuurmann, Max (1889–1955) 57
Schwebsch, Erich (1889–1953) 32f
Senft-Mohr, Emica (1893–1976) 112
Shakespeare, 'Clown's Song' in
 *As You Like It* 108
Sibelius, Jean (1865–1957) 43
silk (for dresses) 108
Simons, Friedel Thomas- *see* Thomas-
 Simons
skeleton 54
Smits, Lory Maier- *see* Maier-Smits
*Song of Initiation* 16, 101
*Soul Calendar* 94, 115
sound, character of 85f
speech eurythmy 24, 34
stage groups 107
Steffen, Albert (1884–1963) 103
Steiner, Marie (1867–1948) 25f, 44,
 106f, 113–15
Stuten, Jan (1890–1948) 44, 112
synecdoche 94

TAO meditation 62f
tetrachord, first (lower) 36, 52, 56
—, second (upper) 36, 52, 56
Thomas-Simons, Friedel (1896–1950)
 22
tone eurythmy 24, 34
— forms 30, 45

tone
—, duration of 72
—, quarter 69
triad 61, 70f
—, major 89
—, minor 89
trochaic rhythm or steps 28f
trousers 107f
*Twelve Moods* 16, 94, 100f

U (*oo*, vowel) 48
uprightness 15

van Deventer-Wolfram, Erna *see*
 Deventer-Wolfram
veils 82, 84f
—, diagonal pinning 110
—, long 110
—, men's 111
—, short 110
—, thick 109
—, thin 109
verbs 99
von Eckhardtstein, Imma *see*
 Eckhardtstein
*Vortakt* 115
vowel(s)
—, concordance sequence 58
—, character of 86f

walking 14
Wigman, Mary (1886–1973) 13
Wolfram, Erna van Deventer- *see*
 Deventer-Wolfram

yellow 86

zodiac 79, 97, 106
—, Egyptian 94
Zuccoli, Elena (1901–96) 44, 79, 115

You may also be interested in...

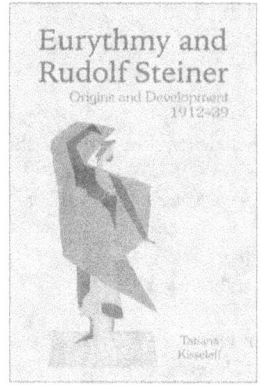
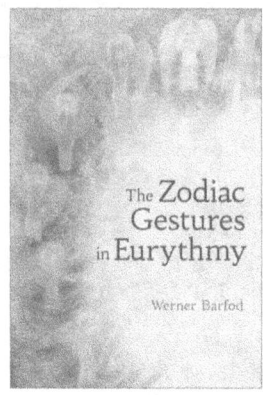
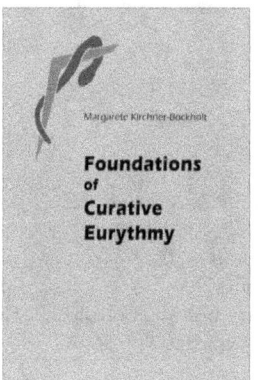
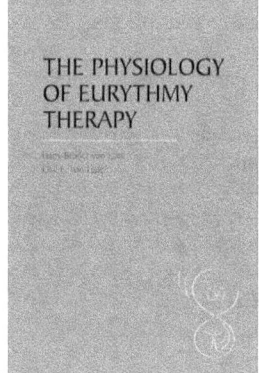

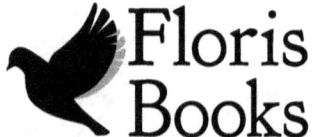

For news on all our **latest books**, and to receive **exclusive discounts, join** our mailing list at: florisbooks.co.uk/signup

*Plus* subscribers get a FREE book with every online order!

*We will never pass your details to anyone else.*

www.ingramcontent.com/pod-product-compliance
Lightning Source LLC
Chambersburg PA
CBHW031228110526
44590CB00035B/3381